Advance Praise

Most Westerners believe that fitness equals good body mechanics: hard muscles, flexible joints, strong lungs, a slow heart rate and low blood pressure. Eastern traditions of self-cultivation such as Qigong, emphasize a different goal: a moving synchrony of body, breath and mind that generates an experience of complete integration. What emerges from such a feeling of natural power is, simply, joy. In *The Way of Joy*, Vicki Dello Joio builds a bridge for us to cross, from East to West, and a way for us to weave together again what has come unraveled—our selves.

—Efrem Korngold, OMD, LAc, co-author of *Between Heaven and Earth,*
  A Guide To Chinese Medicine

For me, *The Way of Joy* is a sacred text. Having studied with Vicki Dello Joio for 13 years, I have learned that out of her deep well of knowledge and wisdom, she has drawn brilliant, utterly fresh insights from which I continually drink, filling me with nourishing waters that flow throughout my life. My study with her is central to my spiritual path; she has taught me to fully embody my spirit, even during years of chronic illness. I already know that my copy of *The Way of Joy* will be underlined, highlighted, dog-eared, and rubbed at the edges—transferred from bedside table to briefcase to backpack, traveling with me every day of my journey. This book reveals the soul of the teacher—like Vicki herself, it is astute and gracious, reverent and funny, crystalline clear and inviting: Pure joy to read and revel in!

—Rev. Dr. Monza Naff, Exec. Dir., Inner Growth Services and Author
  of *Exultation: A Poem Cycle in Celebration of the Seasons*

Vicki and I were both founding members of the Women's Qigong Alliance, an organization dedicated to exploring the challenges of applying ancient Eastern systems in contemporary Western culture, and of doing so as women. Over more than ten years as a student of the *The Way of Joy*, I've found this integrated system to provide a framework for deep inquiry as well as a support for healing. I've been privileged to witness Vicki's embodied masterhood and I'm in awe of how she has integrated her philosophy and practice in this book As you will see, Vicki teaches through her own example, through clear and respectful communication, through beautiful images and stories, and always, always through allowing the wisdom of the practice to illuminate. It's inspiring to see this work rippling out to a wider audience.

—Michele Chase, Chair, Holistic Health Education Graduate Program,
  John F Kennedy University

I have taken *The Way of Joy* with me on my teaching trips across several states and countries, always with the thought in mind that I must share this book with those who can benefit...which is everyone. Written in Vicki's inspiring, expressive voice and filled with enduring Qigong concepts and exercises, you will be taken on a journey of self-inquiry and re-discovery that brings you back to your authentic self. *The Way of Joy* is filled with practical wisdom for anyone on the path of self-mastery. As a master teacher herself, Vicki illuminates "the way" with heart, humor, grit and grace. Her deep understanding of the laws, principles and practices that govern our existence creates a springboard from which to launch our inner and outer explorations. With the skill and intuitiveness of a loving mother knowing her chicks are ready to fly, Vicki gives you a peck on the cheek, a pat on the back and a gentle shove out of your comfort zone, urging you into the unknown to embrace your freedom and your joy with *The Way of Joy* as protection in stormy weather.

— Daisy Lee, Founder of Radiant Lotus Qigong; Advanced Instructor and Clinical Practitioner certified by the National Qigong Association

Vicki Dello Joio is one of those people whose life work is a calling, who can look back and see that she was on her path even before she knew it. She has extensive training from exceptional masters in numerous martial arts, mime, and theater; a deep understanding of Taoist principles; and decades of experience as a gifted master teacher of Chi Kung.

Vicki has integrated this wealth of experience with her own wisdom and created an amazingly intricate, workable system for accessing and using energy as a life force to draw upon, giving us greater power to consciously maximize our potential. She exposes common myths that can hold us in self-defeating, closed circles and shows us, with great clarity, how to find the "pivot point" for moving out of the circle into spirals of growth. Vicki makes it all so accessible, both in how she presents her unique concepts and the practical tools she offers for making life an art, with soul. Having had the privilege of being one of the editors for Vicki's book, I can tell you with absolute confidence, every time I read from the pages of *The Way of Joy*, my life is changed.

—Sharon Strand Ellison, author of *Taking The War Out of Our Words*

The
Way of Joy

An Evolutionary Process to
Awaken Inspiration
Focus Intention
Manifest Fulfillment

Vicki Dello Joio

Wyatt-MacKenzie Publishing, Inc.

The Way of Joy
An Evolutionary Process to Awaken Inspiration, Focus Intention,
Manifest Fulfillment

FIRST EDITION

ISBN:978-0-9820518-9-4
Library of Congress Control Number: 2009928994

Cover and Diagram Design by Sherry Mouser; www.mouserart.com
Layout by Nancy Cleary; www.wymacpublishing.com
Photography by Lois Tema; www.loistema.com

Text set in Berkeley Old Style, Titles in Andalus.

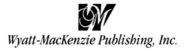

Wyatt-MacKenzie Publishing, Inc.

15115 Highway 36, Deadwood, Oregon 97430
541-964-3314
www.wymacpublishing.com

Dedication

For my Mama, Grayce Dello Joio, whose support and unwavering belief
in me has given me both the foundation and challenge
to deepen in my life and work the explorations of the mysteries
and applications of Joy. Tenacious, curious and courageous,
you have truly been a model for me.

For my life partner, Sherry Mouser, my co-conspirator in Joy,
laughter, and love, my beloved playmate, you are an
unending source of delight and inspiration.

Acknowledgments

Through insights, stories, and love, so many of you—students, friends, colleagues and teachers—are living and breathing through the pages of this book. It exists because of you and my heart is filled with gratitude.

Extra-Special thanks to

Monza Naff, for your brilliant, passionate mentoring of me as a writer, your spiritual guidance, inspired co-visioning, creative mid-wifery, unwavering support, nurturing, and endless editing, and for being a sister of my heart on the sometimes rocky journey of this project.

Sharon Strand Ellison, soul sister, for your generosity of spirit, structural genius, thought-provoking contributions, and profound commitment to this work and our friendship.

Sherry Mouser, for your exquisite artistic vision and renderings, your ceaseless enthusiasm even when creating yet another draft, for thousands of inspiring and fun conversations about joy and for being my heart and soul mate in the mystery.

Khaleghl Quinn, for your luminous teachings so fundamental to my practice and the gift of your love and friendship.

Michele Chase, for your consistent support, enthusiasm, and encouragement as well as for bringing me into the extraordinary graduate program at JFKU.

Judith Cope, for your superb ability to go right to the essence with poetic grace. I could not have asked for a better final editor.

Lois Tema, for your beautiful photography, your light-hearted humor and endurance during the "zen of sitting," and to your skillful and caring assistants, **Laurel Thornton** and **Jackie Yost.**

Living Arts Playback Theater Ensemble, for your consistent, loving support and patience during my long time away.

Nancy Cleary, for your galvanizing, animated and joyful spirit. You truly are a Publisher Extraordinaire.

Ruth Wilson, for your easeful help in redesigning my Chi Kung uniform, your playful humor and your profound embrace of these teachings.

Martha Graham for telling me as a youngster to always follow my heart.

Sparky, for making me laugh along the way. Little four-legged chum, you are truly the living embodiment, great teacher of joy.

Extra Shout-Outs (in alphabetical order by first name) with love and gratitude to Bob Gilbert, Bobby Rothschild, Carol Olwell, Christine Kalb, Chuck Fechner and Susan Lieber, the Combs-Atkinson family, Damaris Jarboux, Donna Belk, Dory Willer, Efrem Korngold, Dr. Garret Yount, the Greenspan family, Jayne Schabel, John Chung, Joyce Lu, Karin Kelly-Givens, Kostas Bagakis, Linda Berry, Lucinda Ramberg, Marcia Kerwitt, Margaret Thompson, Maria Barron, Michael Bell, Michele Chase, Michelle and Merrill, Pat Lane, Rachel Levine-Chernoff, Reba Rose, Rose Berryessa, Ruth Jovel, Sandy Krestan, Stephanie Gertler, Steve Lennon, my brother Justin and mother, Grayce, and all my students, past and present, whose passionate application, challenging questions, and moving stories illuminated my path.

Table of Contents

5. The Walk of Joy   77

Part II The Heart of Joy: Human Triad—Intention   115

6. The Current of Joy   117

7. The Vessel of Joy   131

Note to Reader

To live a joyful life is the greatest accomplishment, and failure
to live joyfully is the greatest loss.
—*Pandit Rajmani Tigunait*

Throughout this book, I refer to "you" (the reader) or to a larger collective "we." While I hope you will feel a resonance with what I am saying, I also imagine there may be times you find yourself thinking, "I don't agree" or "I'm not part of that 'we.'" I want to be clear that in this work I am not espousing one "right" way. I believe that what is most important is that you honor your own wisdom and discernment.

Key Terminology
Some definitions for the terminology you will encounter as you read this book follow:

Chi (also spelled *c'hi, qi*, ji or *ki*): life force, energy, breath, primordial source of all life
Gong work, service, ability
Chi Kung (also spelled *Qigong, Chi Gong, Chi Gung, Ji Gong*, among others): energy work, breath work, meditative, healing, and martial arts from China, based on Taoist principles to cultivate chi. It is sometimes interpreted as Inner Work or Cultivating Life Force
Tai Chi (also spelled *Taiji, T'ai Chi, T'ai Chi-Ch'uan* among others): a martial art sometimes considered to be a style of Chi Kung
Taoism (also spelled *Daoism*): a variety of beliefs and practices based on the study of the Tao (The Way). Originating in China, in essence Taoism is a world-view, "a natural philosophy...based on observation of, and alignment with, the natural and organic nature of things—from planetary movements and the progression of the seasons, to our individual feelings and how they function."[1]

The *Way of Joy* and Chi Kung

My study of Chi Kung, as well as numerous other martial arts, gave me the basis for my understanding of energy and how it works. That understanding, as well as Taoist concepts, serves as the foundation for the Laws, Principles, and Practices I developed into the system I call the *Way of Joy.*

In her comprehensive book, *Breathing Spaces,* Nancy Chen writes "Qigong is a health practice that involves breathing, mental imagery, and sometimes movement. The term 'qigong' has been translated in several ways according to notions of qi as air, breath, energy, or primordial life source."[2] In general, Chi Kung is the name given to a variety of different systems and exercises, both external/physical and internal/meditative, stemming from China and based on Taoist philosophy.

Ranging from guided meditation to gentle slow-moving exercises, all the way to highly athletic, stamina-building forms, Chi Kung is a title as generic as Dance. Just as there are many types of dance (Ballet, Modern, Ballroom, Folk, Tap, etc.), there are many systems of Chi Kung (T'ai Chi Ch'uan, Ba Gua, Iron Shirt, Wild Goose, and so on).

Just as each of those types of dance might be further broken down (modern dance includes the styles of artists like Martha Graham, Merce Cunningham, Pilabolous, etc.), so can many systems of Chi Kung. The martial art Tai Chi, for example, has in itself many different styles and lineages. In fact, "Chi Kung" is a relatively recent name that emerged in China in the '50s as an umbrella term to encompass many forms of exercise geared toward health and healing.

Over the years, I have encountered many different lineages, styles, and practices of Chi Kung. What these systems have in common is that they are all methods of cultivating chi, enhancing the practitioner's ability to work with her or his own life force. As with other types of Oriental medicines, such as acupuncture, Chi Kung is a method with which to direct energy to flow through stagnant areas to create an internal balance.

It's important to me to acknowledge that as a European-American of Italian and Jewish descent, I do not have either historical or biological roots in China or a familial or cultural foundation in Taoism. However, from the time I was a teenager I've had a strong draw to a Taoist worldview and paradigm.

I believe it's imperative to respect and honor the spiritual heritages of these practices. I have studied with a wide range of teachers, from very traditional (including one with whom I was the only white student in a group of all Chinese practitioners) to those with a more Americanized or interpretive approach. To simply superimpose my own interpretation on these lineages would be, I feel, disrespectful.

My intention in naming this system the *Way of Joy* Chi Kung is to honor the traditions that have inspired me and at the same time to acknowledge that this system is a departure from any specific lineage. I would suggest that the freedom to make this work personal is, in its essence, a Taoist approach. As an integrative and interpretative theory and practice, the *Way of Joy* is my offering to the ever-evolving, all-encompassing world-view of Chi Kung and Taoism.

The Way of Joy

PROLOGUE
My Journey to Joy

Inner Joy…isn't the sudden joy of a pleasurable turn of events, it's a constant accompaniment to all activities. Joy arises from within moments of existence, rather than from any other Source.
— David Hawkins

The book you hold in your hands represents a journey that is not only my own but also one I have shared with countless students and clients. The Laws, Principles, and Practices of the *Way of Joy*™ are built on the wisdom of Taoist philosophy and my practice of Chi Kung and other martial arts. At the heart of the system is a focus on how we can access and use the energy of our life force most effectively, while honoring the cycles of our lives, being fully present and embracing all that we experience as food for growth. Whenever I have presented material from the *Way of Joy* in classes, retreats, workshops and speeches, people have invariably asked, "How did you come up with this system?" Here is some of the story of how it came to be.

I have always loved to move. My mother—who was a ballet dancer in New York before she married my father—has told me that even in the crib, whenever I heard music playing, I would haul myself up and, hanging onto the crib rails, bounce in time to the music—always in perfect rhythm, she would add with satisfaction. By the time I was five, I would dance any time I could.

In fact, often when my parents had dinner guests, my father, a composer, would play the piano, and, to my delight, I would be asked to dance for the "company." I felt absolutely free as I was carried on the river of melody with my father's grin beaming over the piano's soundboard, while my mother looked on with pride. Heart filled to bursting, I danced my love of life, leaping and twirling, bringing my hand to my chest as I imagined grasping bouquets of love that I would toss out to shower over all the grown-ups.

During my childhood years, my love of dance translated into a general love of performance, and of theater in particular. In fact, it was through my pursuit of theater that I was first introduced to the martial art of Tai Chi during a summer program for teens at the American

Conservatory Theater in San Francisco. I was immediately drawn to the discipline, grace and beauty of the form, which felt for some inexplicable reason familiar, like something I could almost remember. In subsequent years, as I continued to study T'ai Chi Chuan, I also explored a variety of other martial arts, both internal and external, including Ba Gua, Aikido, Karate, Judo, and the hybrid art, Kajukenbo (which combines Karate, Judo, Jujitzu, Kenpo and Chinese boxing/Kung Fu) as well as Chi Kung.

I loved both the physical challenge and the profound sense of empowerment and focus these arts gave me. In my early 30's I began studying with Chi Kung Master Dr. Khaleghl Quinn.[1] Her brilliant and evocative teachings were instrumental in my development of an even deeper grasp of the meanings held in these ancient patterns of movement. Beyond offering me strength in body and spirit, my practice gave me a greater understanding of myself and my place in the world. I found a way to align with my own sense of purpose. I still remember working out one day when the thought came to me with crystalline clarity, "This is what I am meant to do."

While I had already been teaching Tai Chi for about 20 years, after studying Chi Kung with Dr. Quinn, she encouraged me to teach Chi Kung myself. As I taught specific Chi Kung forms and exercises, I observed and appreciated the impact and transformations that it, other creative and martial arts, and Taoist philosophy brought to my own life and the lives of my students.

I found there was a common heartbeat underlying it all, that quest to embrace a love of life that I did so unerringly as a little dancer of five, where one might move and direct energy from a place of joy and in so doing generate more joy. At that point, I acknowledged that I was no longer teaching any one strict lineage or particular Chi Kung system, but rather was blending and synthesizing a new interpretation and approach for accessing and directing chi.

My process for envisioning and shaping the Way of Joy system has been evolutionary in its progression. I discovered that I had an aptitude for bringing together diverse paths and practices and looking for ways in which the ideas behind them might be interrelated. I looked for, and found, themes that seemed to appear and reappear across diverse arts. I was even able to draw upon my years of training as an actor, mime, and choreographer, my experiments with painting and visual arts, and my explorations through writing. In this way, I formed a coherent system. At yet another level, the Way of Joy seemed to evolve almost by itself.

The Birth of a Name

Musing on my name one day, I realized with a jolt that my birth name, Victoria Dello Joio, when translated from Italian, means Victory of Joy. My initial reaction was "*that's* a daunting legacy. What in the world would it mean to have victory in joy?" My next thought was that my name was a call, something I could try to live up to—to be victoriously joyful beyond any obstacles.

I realized in that moment that I had been carrying a legacy stemming from both of my parents—the love of music I inherited from my father and the love of dance and movement from my mother. Even after I realized that "victory of joy" was a legacy I *wanted* to live up to, it was still many years before I looked back on my whole history and realized it had been, without knowing it, what I had been building toward all my life.

Joy as a Fuel

As my theoretical basis became increasingly more defined, the forms I was practicing and teaching gained ever-greater significance: I realized that each gesture done mindfully revealed a spiritual life lesson. My understanding continued to expand as students asked me questions and I stopped, closed my eyes, and listened inside for the answers. Gradually, I realized that the unifying principle in my work was that Joy could be a fuel for all the choices we make—a fuel instead of an "outcome" of certain choices or mere chance. That insight opened a floodgate of awareness, including the ways in which the practices I had been teaching brought me to this epiphany. From then on, the theory and practice I had been organically evolving not only had a name, the *Way of Joy*, but also became the framework for the refinement of the system I present in this book.

In 1998, at the request of my students, I began offering lecture-seminars. As I spoke and students and other members of my community asked questions, we all reflected on our own life experiences in relation to the themes of each session. Giving those talks further expanded the theoretical basis of what I was teaching. I explored various themes presented in this book—concepts such as "What does it mean to feel joy during excruciating times of pain and loss without just being in denial?" "What is the difference between a boundary and a barrier?" "How can we break open cycles of repeating patterns in our lives and gain new levels of consciousness?"

Ultimately, what emerged became my vision of a set of Laws, Principles, and Practices that fit into the respective concepts of Heaven, Human, and Earth that I had first learned from my earliest studies of Tai Chi and then developed through Dr. Quinn's teaching. Finally, one of my students, a writer and teacher, said, "You're writing a book, you know. You should tape these talks." And so the process of writing began.

We Plan, God Laughs: *An Old Yiddish Saying*

At first I thought I could just take a three-month sabbatical from teaching, live in solitude in the country, and kick-start writing this book. My writer friends laughed and told me that I would need to take at least a year. So I took a deep breath, figured out my finances, and said OK. All I knew was that I needed to take this leap of faith.

But life, as it has a way of doing, intervened. My sabbatical became my challenge—in the face of difficult circumstances, including the severe illness, suffering and death of loved ones—to live out what I teach at the very moment when I wanted to be *writing* what I teach.

Shortly after going off to begin my sabbatical, my beloved uncle telephoned from the East Coast to say he had been diagnosed with end-stage lung cancer, was refusing treatment, and didn't have much time. I flew with my mother, his sister, to Connecticut to be with him during his final journey.

Immediately on my return, a very dear friend and student, Rachel, who was a single mother, was diagnosed with stage three cancer. Two of Rachel's other close friends and I formed teams to organize support for her. Although I did return to the country to write, I continued to work closely with the support teams and had frequent conversations with Rachel about her fears and triumphs.

Just a few months later, my mother, with whom I am very close, was diagnosed with cancer in both breasts. I returned to the Bay Area again to be with her through her procedures and surgery. At one point she and Rachel were in the same hospital on the same floor after surgery, and I found myself running between rooms while one or the other was dozing.

I returned to the country, still keeping close contact with my mother and Rachel, but there were other crises ahead, including holding Rachel's hand when she died, going to be with my partner and her family when her father died, and spending time taking care of my own ailing father on Long Island. It seemed that every time I was back in my writing "groove," I was called away again. Ultimately, as I came close to finishing this book, I spent time with my father during his own process of dying.

There were certainly times when I felt discouraged and overwhelmed, not only by the pain and loss of loved ones, but by the seemingly unending "interruptions" to the writing I felt so driven to do. However, as things progressed, I couldn't help but notice that every time an interruption happened, it crystallized for me the meaning of the very chapter I was working on. Each "detour" contained within it a call to practice that particular theme, as though it was my own Spirit giving me a belt test.[2] I was challenged at every turn to discover and practice how to use the *life force* of joy in the face of severe pain and suffering—my own, and, somehow even more difficult, that of people I loved.

Ultimately it was my practice that carried me through in what I can only call a "state of grace." Not only was I expanding in my commitment of love, but I do believe that I was expanding my spiritual capacity in ways I could never have planned or imagined, enabling me to assert with my whole heart, and with a sense of "kitchen-tested" authority, the principles I am affirming.

My hope is that the concepts and tools in this book will enhance your journey toward conscious living as a fully embodied spirit with a deep sense of purpose, place, and well-being.

CHAPTER 1
The World of Joy

The mystics tell us that when they see what they've been looking at all along but had never seen, they discover an overflowing joy in the heart of things.
— *Anthony de Mello*

When I was a young teen first in love, I remember looking up at the New York City sky. Instead of feeling frustrated and trapped, as I usually did, by the sharp angularity of the tall buildings around me, I was filled with a sense of anticipation, a vision of a full life ahead with endless opportunities and experiences coming my way. I was open and ready to embrace it all, even the eventual loss of this puppy love. In that moment it was life itself I had fallen in love with instead of another 15-year-old whose face I now can barely remember. An internal pulse throbbed through my body, and the gray streets of the city shimmered silver.

Many people associate joy with that kind of romantic feeling of being so in love the whole world looks different. In our goal-oriented society, others believe joy is the reward for doing the right thing, marrying the right person, landing the right job, making enough money. It's the carrot at the end of the stick, the pot at the end of the rainbow. Still others believe joy arrives as a fluke, an accident, a stroke of good fortune that comes unannounced like winning the lottery, being born lucky, or getting rain in the middle of a drought.

What if we take the concept of joy out of the realm of the deserved or undeserved? In this book, I would like to invite you to consider the possibility that joy simply is, that it exists as a mystery inside of us. Like our hearts beating, our breath inhaling and exhaling, joy is part of what keeps us alive whether we pay attention to it or not. If we listen to our hearts beat, we can develop our awareness of an internal rhythm or pulse. If we listen to our breathing, we find that our minds become quieter or increasingly still, that our bodies relax. If we listen deep inside of our psyches for the source of our joy, we will connect to what feels right, even purposeful: a sense of alignment between a Source greater than we are and our own personal expression of that Source. In other words, we begin to feel in balance with the world around us, experience on a visceral level what it means to be one part of the universe, part of the whole. In those moments when we experience a state of joy, as I did as a young innocent embarking into the mysteries of romantic love, we feel at home in the world, happy with the simple reality of being alive and open to all possibilities.

I suggest we look at joy as a fuel that can be accessed in all that we do. Like gasoline in a car, joy is a combustible energy that, when mixed with oxygen (breath), then consumed, can transport us to a new state of being. Or, like a good meal with just the right combination of nutrients (including the nutrient of pleasure) to give our bodies a sense of get-up-and-go, joy can provide us with the sustenance to move towards what we are capable of, to fulfill the potential that we might otherwise shun. When we lose access to that fuel in our lives, we slow down and even stop. Or we substitute other propellants to motivate us, like "shoulds" and "have tos," outside authority, unquestioned habits, social expectations, or simple practicality—"you don't work, you don't get paid." Using these other forms of motivation instead of joy is like using watered-down gasoline, or eating only potato chips for weeks. Our cars might be able to run, or our bodies might continue to function, but in either case we are operating in a diminished way.

When I talk about my work, whether in formal speeches or in casual conversation, I've been struck by how often people look at me, perplexed, and ask, "What is joy anyway? I don't think I've ever felt it." It is as though the feeling has become as elusive as the concept. You might ask yourself what joy is for you. Where does it come from? How do you know when you feel it? Do you ever feel fueled by it?

When I speak of joy, I am not speaking merely of happiness. I don' t mean we never feel sorrow, anger, fear or other difficult emotions. Rather, I envision joy as a container in which all other emotions can be held.[1] In fact, I believe that it is only when we experience all of our emotions, even the painful ones, in relationship to joy that we maintain tranquility, vitality, and our capacity to grow. If we separate painful emotions from the context of joy, they become unbearable, leaving us in despair and turning into a destructive force in our lives.

Therefore I think of joy as a state of being that relishes our full range, the open embrace of all that life brings us, those moments of deep feeling when we know, and can sense, that we are truly alive. This is our birthright. In fact, I believe this state of being is how most of us first experience life. Have you ever watched the delight of an infant as s/he discovers something new, like her toes? For babies who do not suffer abuse, neglect, or other harm, there is a time when every moment is filled with full attention and adventurousness. Even when a baby is angry or frustrated, sad or simply hungry, s/he fully embraces all of the feelings of each moment. A friend told me that once, upon holding a newborn for the first time, he exclaimed that she looked like a baby Buddha. The midwife smiled as she took the baby back and said that all babies are born baby Buddhas.

I believe for many of us joy frequently flashes its brilliance, yet too often we take it for granted, are too preoccupied to notice it, or forget the experience as soon as it passes. Perhaps it occurs with the scent of the season's first ripe strawberry as you raise it to your lips. Perhaps it's in a sigh of deep satisfaction when you first lie down in bed after a good day's hard work. Perhaps it's in the first glimpse of inspiration in your fantasies of a creative project you would dearly love to take on. Or perhaps it's sparked by a special work of art, a song on the radio, or a walk among the redwoods.

But we touch our joy in many more ways than in the realm of the unexpected and easily forgotten. There are times when you might have found yourself taking a more pro-active, if unintentional, approach to experience joy. Even though you might not have been aware of it as a driving force, you may have been fueled by it. For instance, joy lives in the world of "just because." Have you ever just gone out and stood still in a downpour? Called an old friend "just because"? Written a poem and put it on the refrigerator? Doodled a sketch you didn't want to throw away? Taken a spontaneous trip to a museum or a matinée movie—all instead of doing what you were "supposed to do"? I think all of these activities are an instinctive call, an invitation back to our birthright: a feeling of enjoyment ("in-joy-meant" or "meant to be in joy") that we once knew as a moment-to-moment reality.

When we go one step further and take the time to acknowledge our joy, it tends to replenish itself, become more available and abundant. Unlike gas or food, I believe our joy is a limitless wellspring: the more you use it, the more there is to use. Self-replenishing, like a spring bubbling up from its source, it can pervade our lives, our sense of purpose, our place in the world, just as water moves from springs to creeks to rivers into the ocean. And I believe that this limitless wellspring is always available to us for inspiration, creation, and motivation. I believe joy lives in our essence, our *chi*, in the space and in the particles of aliveness that unite all living beings and that it is expressed differently through the uniqueness of each one.

A musician friend once spoke to me about how music and rhythms vibrate in us and around us all the time. We just need to tap into the right frequency to hear them. I think it is the same with joy. As we draw it from our internal experience, joy is often mirrored back by our environment. Have you ever had a day where things just fell into place, went right for you, and when you walked out into the street radiating that feeling encountered, to your surprise, a stranger who smiled at you and said hello? Joy can be contagious. At other times, rather than simply mirroring our mood, the environment may stimulate a change in us. As a different example, a friend told me her mood for the entire day brightened when, on her way to work, she noticed a small flowering plant pushing up through the concrete on the side of the freeway. She said she'd find herself smiling suddenly as she went through the mundane routines of her day.

I would also suggest that joy can be not only the container for all other emotions, even those perceived as negative or draining, it can be the foundation for them as well. While we can feel anger or grief when our joy has been depleted, or we have forgotten it's there, I also see anger, even rage, as the warrior/protector of joy, erupting when our sense of what is right, fair, or just, is threatened.

Likewise, I believe joy is at the source of feelings of tragedy or loss. For instance, I've experienced several beloved friends dying of cancer or AIDS. Even facing such irreparable loss, I have found myself and others in an exalted state of being, combining sobs with laughter at a memory, experiencing a sense of celebration of that individual's life and gifts at the same time as mourning the absence of their physical being. Without the remembered joy, there would be no sorrow.

There have been times when I was teaching a class when a student was going through a difficult emotion or particular challenge. When I related it to a Taoist seasonal interpretation or a principle from the Way of Joy, I would see that student sigh in relief as her or his body dropped into a more relaxed and comfortable posture. I think there was something about sensing an interconnectedness between a personal experience and something larger than self, be it a season or energetic principle, that allowed that individual to feel in a deeply personal way that their particular challenge was not just an isolated phenomenon. This produced a type of relaxation I sometimes think of as the "joy slump." Being part of a greater whole, sensing in a personal way that we are not separate, that we are, in fact, integrated into a larger fabric or energetic community, offers more than relief. I believe it also connects us to the source of joy.

To summarize, I define joy as the ability to live life wholly in its abundance, including the full expression of all other emotions. While I think many of us have been trained to see it as a consequence of our actions, I believe that if we take our joy as a starting place, we'll not only have more fun, we'll be better able to experience life more fully, attain our goals, move toward our destiny. If a willingness, even eagerness, to experience the whole of our lives were the starting place for every choice we made, what would our lives look like? What might we begin to develop for ourselves and our communities? What if joy, a deep embrace of all that faces us, were the motivation to get up in the morning, instead of forcing ourselves out of bed because of obligation?

Because we live in a world so out of balance, it might seem almost inconceivable, I know. Nevertheless, I believe we are capable of interpreting our experiences, evolving our responses, and cultivating an ability to make our own choices with consciousness. How might we develop an awareness of joy on every level—physical, emotional, mental, and spiritual? What tools can we use to express our particular uniqueness? And, finally, how might we experience the connective tissue, our interrelationships, with all living beings, and so invite recognition, an ever-present living awareness of our place in the web of life? This book provides a set of Laws, Principles, and Practices that can guide us. Using them, we can access what I believe we were put on the planet to experience, to remember what we knew as enlightened baby Buddhas.

CHAPTER 2

The Shape of Joy

Three Realms of Consciousness
Heaven, Human and Earth

The hair on our bodies raises, almost like antennae, to connect
with something greater, larger than our daily lives.
A sense of promise, magic, mystery and unutterable beauty.
—*Vicki Dello Joio*

When I was that young teen in love and the grey streets of New York seemed to shimmer silver, it was my love that made everything around me look different. Sometimes an experience like that can change us for life; other times, the streets soon turn grey again.

Many years later, in 1985, I had an experience that *did* change me forever. I was in Germany, in my mid-thirties, where I was touring and performing with Common Threads, a women's theater company I had co-founded.

While in Europe, I met with an old friend, another martial artist, who told me about a teacher named Wolfgang[1] who lived in a small town in southern Germany. She told me he had extraordinary powers and urged me to come visit her there, to see for myself the things he could do.

Wolfgang had an ability to understand how energy works in ways I had never seen before. What I saw surprised and dismayed me. I witnessed him using energy as a force to manipulate others employing methods that were previously beyond my comprehension. Even now, I often hesitate to tell the story for fear of losing credibility—the kind of story that we describe as "impossible" to believe.

While I will tell the complete story later as an example of the Principle, *Integrity Activates Change*, what I want to emphasize here is that watching Wolfgang use his chi (energy) dramatically expanded my consciousness about what is possible. I watched the "impossible" instantly become reality. My understanding of human potential, of life itself, changed forever. I believe many of us have had some version of this type of experience. We may be afraid to talk about it for the very reason I mentioned, fear of how others will respond—how they will regard us for claiming something to be true that seems so outrageous.

These experiences can become our "best kept secrets." It may be something as dramatic as a near-death experience, or a deceased loved one appearing in some form. It may be something utterly simple, such as gaining a newfound appreciation of the stages of life while holding a newborn baby. Once we have had an experience that alters our consciousness, it's almost impossible to turn back.

What I witnessed awakened me to what was possible in how we can use energy. Instead of one man or certain isolated persons using their chi to gain personal power, I wondered, 'How might we access this energy to shift consciousness and enhance life for all?' The walls of what I had thought of as "reality" had been shattered and I found myself in a new universe. This awakening thrust me into a world with far more mystery and potential than I could have imagined.

An Introduction to the Three Realms

Throughout my journey of exploring the themes of Taoism through Chi Kung, I have encountered critical junctures through which I learned profound lessons about the nature and function of what I call the "Three Realms of Consciousness"—Heaven, Human, and Earth. These three realms relate to three energy centers called the triple *tan tien,* which are also referred to as the triple warmer or triple heater in Traditional Chinese Medicine (TCM). They are primary energy centers for our connection to the universe and our experience in life. How we access and use the energy in each of these realms constitutes the basis for much of Chi Kung. In short, the Heaven realm contains consciousness and inspiration, the Human realm contains intention and love, and the Earth realm is empowerment and manifestation.

Despite how misguided I believe Wolfgang was, I came out with an expanded awareness of what I would call the Heaven realm—where what I had thought could only exist in my imagination became real. I felt called upon to discover how I could use this emerging consciousness to not only cultivate inner strength in myself, but also to tap its potential for empowering an entire community and beyond.

Before going to Europe I had been training in Kajukenbo.[2] Having been physically attacked on the street, I had begun studying some of the "hard" martial arts to become safer. When I returned to the United States from Europe, I resumed my Kajukenbo training with my Sifu (teacher), Professor Coleen Gragen.

While I loved the training and the innovative, empowering teachings of my Sifu, I found myself focusing on how I might cultivate my own chi in ways informed by what I had seen in Germany. Disenchanted with the idea of relying on physical prowess as my sole means of protection, I searched for ways I could apply what I had seen in order to protect myself without fighting. This process of personalizing inspiration is a property of the Human realm where you take the impetus from the Heaven realm and translate it to make it work in your own life.

A few months after I returned from Europe, I had a different kind of street experience. I could see that a man walking toward me intended to grab me. In that encounter, I found myself intuitively using chi to deflect an attack in a way that involved no physical contact. I was able to protect myself without using a physical form of self-defense. This literal action—happening in real time and incorporating a new and empowered way of being—is the property of the Earth realm. Using chi in this way was a direct *application* of my own *translation* of the *inspiration* I found in Germany.

After stretching my ideas of what was "real" in my encounter with Wolfgang (Heaven realm), I began to think about how to personally integrate that information in my own life (Human realm). By the time that next attack on the street came, I turned what I had been working to conceptualize into an actual spontaneous response (Earth realm).

There is an intricate relationship between all three realms. The Human realm functions to bring the Heaven realm and the Earth realm together. How we use energy in the Human realm facilitates a relationship between inspiration (Heaven) and behavior (Earth). While functioning in the Human realm, not only have we translated inspiration into practical experience, but the way we respond in the moment has been elevated toward the ideals that inspire us.

The relationships among all three realms are fluid. Each time we make a change in one realm, the other two realms are impacted. The street incident prompted me to let go of the training I was doing in all other forms of martial arts. For several years, I studied Chi Kung with Master Teacher Dr. Khaleghl Quinn, and over time cultivated a discipline in which I practiced many hours a day.

On March 28, 1990, a car going about 30 miles an hour hit me as I was crossing the street. Although I was thrown quite a distance, I landed in a martial arts roll and was not seriously injured. Soon after, having been taken by ambulance to San Francisco General Hospital, I remember hearing doctors and nurses discussing how it seemed miraculous that I had not broken anything, or been killed, even, by the double impact of the car striking me and my landing on the concrete.

Since the first incident on the street, my work to develop and integrate all three realms had strengthened my chi in remarkable ways. Through my practice I had supported my *jing*—the actual physical life force or stamina in my body—to such a degree that I could survive an accident of some magnitude and walk away relatively unscathed.

Let's look now in more depth at how each of these realms functions.

Heaven Realm

The spirit down here in man and the spirit up there in the sun, in reality are only one spirit, and there is no other one.
—*Upanishads*

Have you ever lain on your back and gazed at the night sky dotted with stars and planets, marveling at all the pinpricks of starlight in the velvety blackness of space?

On a solo camping retreat in the mountains, I decide to sleep outside of my tent. As I lie on the ground looking up, I'm filled with a rush of awareness, my body conscious of being so very small, an atom, perhaps, on this planet, which itself, I realize, is merely a molecule in the vastness of space. I've never felt so tiny. At the same time, I can sense that my entire physical being is made up of cells, molecules, atoms from the very marrow of my bones to each hair on my skin. I feel as though my body itself is a universe containing a vast number of small worlds. So at the same time as I experience myself as minuscule in relation to the universe, I also experience myself as immense, containing an entire universe within.

The Heaven realm is expansive. It sparks us to travel to new levels of awareness, inspires and guides us to set off on uncharted paths. When I speak of Heaven, I am not referring to a post-mortem destination, but rather to a level of consciousness or awareness that we can choose to tap into or not.

Here we are able to envision what might be possible in our world and in our lives. Corresponding to the first hexagram of the I Ching—"The Creative" ☰ made up of all *yang* or unbroken lines—the Heaven realm relates to your vision, your imagination and your inspiration. It's the home to your muse, where the experience of "aha!" lives, where ideas appear spontaneously.

The *yang* of Heaven is expressive, expansive, and active. It instigates change. Consider, for example, how the moon influences ocean tides, how the sun and rain impact life on earth. In the same way, the yang energy of the Heaven realm influences us, changes our awareness, our consciousness within the very cells of our bodies.

In Chi Kung, the energy of heaven has been described as being accessed through a funnel-like shape that points down towards the crown of the head and resonates in the space three feet above the head, in the head and in the neck. Located around the pineal gland in the brain in the upper *tan tien*, this energy center is called *Shen* (Spirit). The Heaven realm is where we connect to Source or God/Goddess, to our spirituality. Here lies the "We-Are-All-One" consciousness, where there is no separation between self and other, what mystics have called the One Self, One Mind. Mystics also refer to the Witness, or the Observer Self. Our Observer Self just is. A neutral presence outside time and space, neither reactive nor judgmental, when we tap into it, we access universal wisdom and gain insight and inspiration.

Whether you place this concept of heaven in a religious/spiritual context (i.e., God(s), Goddess(es), Divine Intervention, Higher Power, the Angelic Realm, etc.) or in a material/scientific one (the exploration of the macrocosm that is our vast and unexplored universe) or both, the Heaven realm brings 1) an awareness of and 2) access to that which is greater than the individual self. Here you might imagine yourself in outer space, yet able, with an eagle's clear vision, to view your life on this planet as being as small as an ant colony.

Heaven thus represents our wisdom, our minds at full potential. It refers to the enormous unused capacity of our brains and bodies. This is the level of being where we see the whole picture, expand our consciousness, hold the large perspective, experience "Oneness." It is the world of infinite possibilities, where everything we can imagine is real, or has the possibility of becoming manifest.

Human Realm

Our own life is the instrument with which we experiment with Truth.
—*Thich Nhat Hanh*

Have you ever been inspired to create something, then become intimidated by its vastness? Have you felt as though you haven't known how to sustain the largeness of your vision when you began to implement it? Did you then find as you began to limit the scope of your vision, you were able to focus on the formation, the process of bringing that vision to life?

Staring at a large canvas covered haphazardly with pieces of red and yellow tissue paper, I am filled with despair. Wanting to create the image of fire in the next piece in my collage series on the four elements, I've schlepped paper, paints, tissue paper, pastels, pencils and other art supplies out to this small cabin in the woods outside of Garberville. I have even invested in an easel, somewhat abashedly since I do not think of myself as a visual artist. The time has arrived.

Quiet days of solitude stretch out in front of me. I feel completely over-whelmed, inadequate and hopeless. "What makes you think you can do justice to the experience of fire? It's too vast, too consuming!" I mutter as I pace in circles. I am livid, furious at myself, enraged at fire. I squat in front of the pot-bellied stove that is providing warmth on this cold wintry morning and stare into it morosely. I sigh. I pace, I squat, I sigh.

My eyes fall on a little pile of ash that has gathered toward the front of the stove's basin. Hopelessly I scoop it onto a finger, rubbing the grit with my thumb. I turn to the canvas and smear a blackened streak on the bottom left corner of the paper. I stand back, sighing yet again. "It makes a little sense," I think. I get more ash and add a couple of blackened twigs. Before I know it, it is the end of the day and that bottom left corner finally feels right.

As the days go by, the corner expands to create a foundation for the painting that gradually rises up into an image of flame. I feel enthralled, heated to my core.

In the Human realm, we narrow the picture down so it is manageable, so we have a starting point to make something real. Only when we make the Heaven-based vision initially smaller, more attainable, can the Human realm become home to joy, where we co-create our lives with Source. While the Heaven realm contains Wisdom, it is in the Human realm where we formulate that information into something we can work with and express. Heaven penetrates our consciousness with wisdom, guidance and inspiration; our hearts respond. When we are inspired by Source (Heaven), we experience our interconnectedness, our Love, and our joy (Human). Joy is the activating principle that enables us to take what is universal and discover how to act on it in a way that is personal.

Each of us has a unique way of bringing forth what inspires us. You might say that in the Heaven realm, we are all one, all part of a great Cosmic gem. In the Human realm, we are each a single facet on that gem that expresses universality in a unique way according to culture, beliefs, background, talent, values, personality, and so on.

According to Taoist thought, humans live between Heaven and Earth. Located in the middle *tan tien* (energy center) in the torso between the neck and navel with the heart at its center, the human realm in Chi Kung is referred to as *Tai*, or as *Taiji*. In the I Ching, *T'ai* (Peace) is the eleventh hexagram and is symbolized by the reversal of heaven and earth. ☷ The trigram for earth ☷, depicted by three open or *yin* lines, is above. The trigram for heaven ☰ depicted by three solid or *yang* lines, is below. As humans, it is our place and responsibility within this alignment to draw heaven down to manifest here on earth and simultaneously to raise the energy of earth up to meet heaven. The energy of the polarity of this simultaneous up and down movement ripples out into wider and wider concentric circles of influence and interdependence, connecting us to the web of life.

Thus the Human realm is the area of communication, where we experience ourselves in relationship to one another and to the world around us: people, places, animals, the earth, all other living beings. Here we discover, honor, and work with both our own uniqueness and with the rich diversity we have among us as humans and as one of the species on this planet.

At the same time, the Human realm is also where we are called upon to work with limitations. When we're still in the Heaven realm, or in a visionary, inspired state, everything seems possible. When we look up at the sky, however, we cannot see the whole sky at one time. We can only perceive as far as our eyes can see—our ability to take it in is limited. So too, when we're in the experience of day-to-day existence, the vastness of our full potential is far greater than we can conceive. We're unable to comprehend it in its entirety. A poem by Emily Dickenson contains the line, "The truth dazzles gradually or else the whole world would be blind." In other words, for humans to try to take in the vastness of the Heavens would only "blind" us with overwhelming brightness.

Thus, Heaven is available to us only in glimpses, can only be accessed a little at a time. It is in the Human realm that we take those glimpses or flashes of insight and begin to work with our limits, deal with the details, create a plan. You might look at this as first having the vision of the house you want to build and then creating blueprints that fit the limits of your budget. It is here in the Human realm that we face both the setbacks and the challenges of discovering "how to."

When faced with the limits embedded in the Human stage, people often "lose heart" and disconnect from joy. As individuals with different values, different styles of learning and being, different degrees of tolerance for discomfort, we make choices every day about how to follow through (or not) on our vision. As Wayne Dyer says in *The Power of Intention*, "Free will

means that you have the choice to connect to spirit or not."[3] When difficulties arise, when realizing a dream is not as easy as it may have seemed,
you might find yourself becoming discouraged or wanting to give up. The
Human realm is what pessimists (who think of themselves as realists) call
the "real world," where we bump into the challenges that make us stop,
pause, face our own uncertainties, doubts and demons. "How am I gonna
do this when I can't even pay off my car?" "I've got this great idea, but
everyone keeps saying I'm crazy, it's impossible. They're probably right."
When we bump into these obstacles, we're given the opportunity to renew
our choices about inner direction, to discern what feeds us and what drains
us, to work realistically within our limitations without giving up the dream.

In the Human realm you are called upon to strengthen your commitment, to forge your intention, to reengage with both your inspiration born
in the Heaven realm with what motivates you to begin with—your passion,
your heart, your joy. In fact, you can experience the Human realm as the
place to use, even celebrate, limitations.

I believe that this is true even for people who create mostly out of
pain, loss or confusion. They may find that working within their limitations
can ultimately offer release and transformation. For example, when I was
working on the fire collage and I thought about fire in general, I became
overwhelmed. I had already created a collage of water for a series on the
four elements. As I conceived of my image for fire, I thought it would be
easy, that it would just burn itself onto the page. I was dismayed to discover
the enormity of the subject and became overwhelmed and discouraged. It
was only when I began to limit my scope of vision and focus on the small
details that I could begin to build the larger image. It was in looking
through the *limits* of "how to" that I created the piece. And by limiting
myself to specifics I was able to turn work into play, stagnation into flow.

So the Human realm is both powerful (in that it channels the vision
of heaven) and challenging (in that it becomes denser or harder to follow
through toward our vision or sometimes even to believe in it). Whether we
are creating a piece of art or the texture of our lives, joy is the glue that
holds that power and that challenge.

Earth Realm

*The sun shines not on us, but in us. The rivers flow not past, but through us, thrilling
tingling, tingling, vibrating every fiber and cell of the substance of our bodies, making
them glide and sing.*
—John Muir

Have you ever had a dream of something you would like to have or do and then experienced a synchronistic flow of events that led to its realization?

I enter the rental house through the back door and follow the landlord up the back stairs, barely registering the information he is droning out in wheezy puffs. As I walk onto the small landing outside of the back door, I am thrown by the sweet scent of lemon blossoms. I stand very still gulping in deep breaths.

As a child growing up in a city, I had a recurring dream, one that I may have gotten from a movie: I was living in a place where I could walk onto a back porch and pluck a lemon from a tree. The image had become a symbol of a place I wanted to live someday, a state of being I was yearning for.

I gaze at the cluster of bright yellow orbs next to my shoulder, then tear myself away to follow the landlord into a spacious living room large enough, I recognize in a flash, for me to teach Chi Kung classes. It feels as though this house has come to me out of the blue, the result of a casual comment I had made in class a few weeks earlier—that I no longer wanted to live in San Francisco. This house subsequently became both my home and the launching pad for the Way of Joy *school.*

Anytime we manifest a dream, we are operating on the Earth realm. This is where we bring the vision inspired in the Heaven realm, formed and shaped by the Human realm, into actual manifestation. Here is the matter, the material substance of what we first envisioned, the destination of Heaven.

The Earth is our foundation. It's both literally the ground we stand on and figuratively where we "stand our ground," where we experience solidity in who and what we are, feel our place in the universe. From this plane we draw the strength, stability, and confidence to make our dreams materialize, to live our convictions, to walk our talk.

This is the clay we have to work with—malleable and affected by our intention—in the same way, as I described earlier, that the earth is impacted by the sun and moon, indeed by the cosmos. In the I Ching, the Earth realm corresponds to the second hexagram, "The Receptive." ☷ This hexagram is made up of all *yin* lines, responsive and open to change.

The Earth realm in Chi Kung is called *Jing*. Located in the lower *tan tien* (energy center) in the hips, pelvis, legs, and feet, *jing* extends three feet down into the earth. Energetically shaped like a pyramid, with the top pointing up towards the heart, the Earth realm is home to our corporeal being, the actual matter of which our bodies are made.

This realm is the source of our health and our wealth, the place our nourishment comes from, both literally and symbolically. This plane also holds physical and narrative histories, whatever has formed you, made you the person you are, as well as the strength and knowledge that come from your ancestors, roots, and heritages both biological and spiritual.

Because it contains the past, the Earth realm also includes the underground (what lies beneath the surface), where your unconscious influences you, your dream world informs you. This is sometimes confusing to people because dreams can also be a source of inspiration. However, I am referring here to images that arise from the unconscious, ones that may be surprising, disturbing or simply impressionistic, and that influence us in ways we may not be clear about. I am distinguishing this kind of dream from the "aha!" visionary flash of inspiration characterized by the Heaven realm.

The Earth realm is where "composting"[4] happens, where we have the opportunity to transform our experiences, turn waste into fertilizer. Here, pain, difficulties and trauma, as well as outdated conditioning from the past, have the potential to become food for strength instead of a weakness that siphons off our life force.

Take, for example, the case of Jerome, an ex-con who had been the victim of severe abuse and neglect as a child. He had been busted for drug-related crimes when he was a young adult. As he was developing a strong spiritual awareness, he discovered his calling and became a counselor for inner city youth. Jerome inspired and improved the lives of many around him. In other words, it was through his own spiritual development, his access to the Heaven realm, that he was able to transform his past and take positive action in his life on the Earth realm.

When we draw the breath of Heaven (Inspiration) down to Earth, as Jerome did, we aerate the soil and accelerate the composting. This is how the Heaven realm illuminates the Earth realm in our Human experience. Light shines on the shadows, on what has been hidden. Heaven is ethereal and light, the place of full potential where anything is possible. The Human realm is denser and where we take heart to move through challenges. The Earth realm, the densest of all three levels, is where we are at our most "concrete," where making things happen is hardest, where any remaining resistance must be faced and overcome. This is the final stage of hard labor in the birth of a project or intention, the final exertion of will, of pushing. The result is Creation Manifest.

Way of Joy: Laws, Principles and Practices

As I have worked with and mused on the Heaven, Human and Earth realms over the years, I've thought about them in the context of a full-hearted embrace of all-that-is. This has given birth to the *Way of Joy*, the theory and practice I have developed. Because it is a personal expression of my own understanding of some fundamental Taoist tenets, I would say it is my own Human realm work. That is, what you are reading is my own understanding, interpretation, and personal application of these three realms.

In the *Way of Joy*, the Heaven realm has three inherent "Laws," the Human realm has three inherent "Principles," and the Earth realm has three inherent "Practices." In essence, the *Way of Joy* Laws (Heaven realm) are *universal* theories, the Principles (Human realm) are the ways in which you *personally interpret* those theories, and the Practices (Earth realm) are the *embodiment* of how to apply that theoretical understanding in your daily life.

Heaven Realm: Laws

When I refer to a *Way of Joy* "Law," I don't mean these are rules of conduct you are supposed to follow. Rather, I'm using the word in the way science might refer to a Law—as in the Law of Gravity or the Laws of Physics. These are energetic concepts, premises that are universal or constant, and so are part of the Heaven realm. The three *Way of Joy* Laws of energy in the Heaven Realm are:

- *Within Motion, Stillness; Within Stillness, Motion*
- *Chi Moves in the Space Between*
- *Circles Open into Spirals*

These Laws of the Heaven realm invoke our *awareness* and give the spiritual context or broad overview for the three Principles we can use to guide us in the Human realm.

Human Realm: Principles

As properties of the Human realm, the *Way of Joy* Principles refer to the ways in which you might experience, interpret or express the Heaven realm Laws in your own life. Here the Laws become personal to you. They are interpreted by you and so inform and influence your choices according to your values. When these Principles are aligned with the Laws, you create a flow that contains the elements of how to live your intention in a meaningful way. To again quote Wayne Dyer in *The Power of Intention*, "The moments of your life, which you spend being happy and joyful and allowing yourself to be fully alive and on purpose, are the times you are aligned with the all-creating universal mind of intention."[5]

The three *Way of Joy* Principles I describe as properties of the Human realm are:

- *Balance Brings Harmony*
- *Boundaries Dissolve Barriers*
- *Integrity Activates Change*

These Principles can guide you as you shape the concepts of the universal Laws (Heaven) into the values and tools that fuel your *intention* about what you apply to your life experience.

Earth Realm: Practices

The three Practices of the *Way of Joy* contain a range of Chi Kung forms and other exercises, tools to use to "walk your talk," make the Principles of the Human realm concrete and manifest. They keep the Principles vibrant and accessible in specific ways. The very names of each Practice are themselves key directives to a particular attitude or approach. Providing ways to embody the inspiration of the Laws and apply the Principles, the three *Way of Joy* Practices in the Earth Realm are:

- *Embrace Wholeness*
- *Cultivate Discernment*
- *Allow Alchemy*

The specific Practices contain prompts and exercises you can use from day to day and situation to situation to keep yourself aligned with both your source/wisdom (Heaven) and your joy (Human) so that you are *empowered* (Earth) to manifest your heart's desire.

Way of Joy Triads

The Laws, Principles and Practices do not function only within their own realm. Each of the Three Realms of Consciousness contains a triad consisting of one Law (Heaven), one Principle (Human), and one Practice (Earth). Thus, each realm contains one element from each of the other realms.

The **Heaven triad** consists of the first Law—or universal theory—*Within Motion, Stillness; Within Stillness, Motion,* the first Principle—or way to personalize the Law—*Balance Brings Harmony;* and the first Practice—what you actually do to walk the talk of this triad—*Embrace Wholeness.*

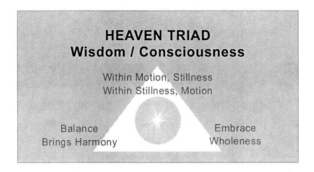

The **Human triad** consists of the second Law, *Chi Moves in the Space Between*, the second Principle, *Boundaries Dissolve Barriers*, and the second Practice, *Cultivate Discernment*.

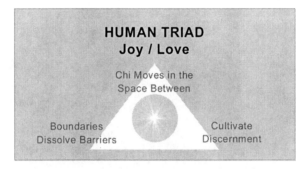

The **Earth triad** consists of the third Law, *Circles Open into Spirals*, third Principle, *Integrity Activates Change*, and third Practice, *Allow Alchemy*.

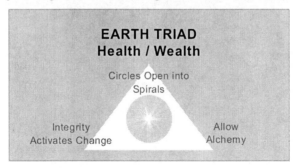

Because each *triad*—Heaven, Human and Earth—contains within it aspects of the other *realms*, it may be easy to get confused. It will be helpful to remember that the Laws *always* represent Heaven, the Principles *always* represent Human, and the Practices *always* represent Earth, regardless of which triad they appear in. Please see the three charts on the following pages for visual representations of the workings of these realms and triads.[6]

In the following chapters, as I present the *Way of Joy*, I hope you will explore and deepen your own reflections on the workings of the three realms—Heaven, Human and Earth—in your life. When we ignore them, we create blocks for ourselves. On the other hand, when we understand the workings of these realms and the interrelations among them, we can intentionally create a path toward manifestation and fulfillment that infuses our lives with the embodiment of Spirit and Joy.

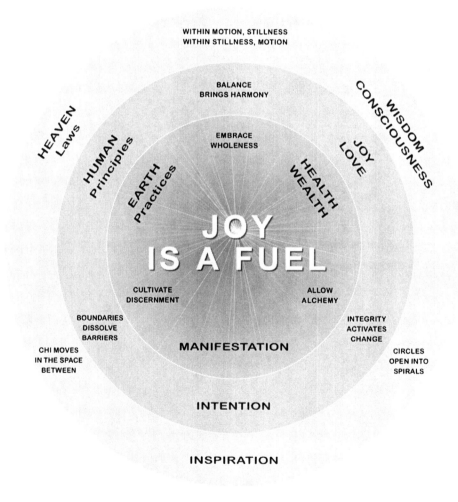

WITHIN MOTION, STILLNESS
WITHIN STILLNESS, MOTION

BALANCE
BRINGS HARMONY

EMBRACE
WHOLENESS

HEAVEN Laws

HUMAN Principles

EARTH Practices

WISDOM CONSCIOUSNESS

JOY LOVE

HEALTH WEALTH

JOY IS A FUEL

CULTIVATE
DISCERNMENT

ALLOW
ALCHEMY

BOUNDARIES
DISSOLVE
BARRIERS

INTEGRITY
ACTIVATES
CHANGE

CHI MOVES
IN THE SPACE
BETWEEN

CIRCLES
OPEN INTO
SPIRALS

MANIFESTATION

INTENTION

INSPIRATION

Way of Joy Chi Kung™

CHART 1

	HEAVEN	HUMAN	EARTH
I Ching Hexagrams	CH'IEN The Creative	T'AI Peace	K'UN The Receptive
Primary Associations	HEAVEN TRIAD Wisdom / Consciousness Within Motion, Stillness Within Stillness, Motion Embrace Wholeness Balance Brings Harmony	HUMAN TRIAD Joy / Love Chi Moves in the Space Between Cultivate Discernment Boundaries Dissolve Barriers	EARTH TRIAD Health / Wealth Circles Open into Spirals Allow Alchemy Integrity Activates Change
Fundamentals	**LAWS** Within Motion, Stillness Within Stillness, Motion Chi Moves in the Space Between Circles Open into Spirals	**PRINCIPLES** Balance Brings Harmony Boundaries Dissolve Barriers Integrity Activates Change	**PRACTICES** Embrace Wholeness Cultivate Discernment Allow Alchemy
	HEAVEN	HUMAN	EARTH

Way of Joy Chi Kung™

CHART 2

HEAVEN

Shen
Upper Tan Tien

*Head, Neck
and Three Feet
Above Head*

Inspiration
Wisdom
Consciousness
Perspective
Cosmos
Source
Destiny
Illumination
Vision
Intuition
Potential
Infinite Possibilities

Yang

LAWS

Within Stillness, Motion;
Within Motion, Stillness
Chi Moves in the Space Between
Circles Open into Spirals

HEAVEN TRIAD

Within Motion, Stillness
Within Stillness, Motion

Balance
Brings Harmony

Embrace
Wholeness

HUMAN

T'ai
Middle Tan Tien

*Base of Throat (Thymus)
Heart & Solar Plexus*

Intention
Joy
Love
Compassion
Self-knowledge
Individuality
Personal Expression
Uniqueness
Communication
Relationships
Connections
Interdependence

Balance
Yin/Yang

PRINCIPLES

Balance Brings Harmony
Boundaries Dissolve Barriers
Integrity Activates Change

HUMAN TRIAD

Chi Moves in the
Space Between

Boundaries
Dissolve Barriers

Cultivate
Discernment

EARTH

Jing
Lower Tan Tien

*Hips, Legs, Feet and
Three Feet
Into the Ground*

Manifestation
Health
Wealth
Empowerment
Nourishment
Creativity
Grounding
Instinct
Dreams (unconscious)
Spiritual and
Biological Heritages
Transformation

Yin

PRACTICES

Embrace Wholeness
Cultivate Discernment
Allow Alchemy

EARTH TRIAD

Circles Open
into Spirals

Integrity
Activates Change

Allow
Alchemy

Way of Joy Chi Kung™

PART I

The Spirit of Joy
Inspiration

HEAVEN TRIAD
Wisdom / Consciousness

Within Motion, Stillness
Within Stillness, Motion

Balance   Embrace
Brings Harmony   Wholeness

As long as we remain closed to the possibility of spiritual help in our unfolding,
we are choosing to operate off the battery pack of our limited resources.
When we are open to spiritual assistance—however tentatively, however
experimentally—we tap into unlimited supply.
—Julia Cameron

The Heaven triad of the *Way of Joy* contains the Law, Principle, and Practice that provide the inspiration and vision for the other two triads. I begin with the Heaven realm so that we may comprehend and experience more fully the direction of chi as it flows from the Heaven realm (inspiration), through the Human realm (interpretation), to the Earth realm (manifestation). However, as you delve more deeply into the substance of these ideas, you will find you can experience each realm (and its interplay with the other two) by entering at any level, because ultimately, as you can see in Chart 1, p. 37, the construct is actually a circle.

Located in the neck, head, and three feet above the head, and drawing from the crown chakra, the Heaven realm is the receptor for receiving wisdom from universal consciousness. The question is—how do we access this wisdom from that Source? Some find their access though prayer, others through meditation, while still others through Yoga or Chi Kung. What are the ways in which *you* access Spirit, draw from the expansive perspective of the Cosmos, your experience of "Aha!"?

    I believe whatever method we use has a common thread, illuminated by the Law of the Heaven triad: *Within Motion, Stillness; Within Stillness, Motion.* Have you ever been stopped in your tracks by the sound of the wind singing though the trees and for that one moment nothing else existed? Within the motion of the sound you become utterly still (within motion, stillness). And at the core of your stillness, you tune in and respond to the sound of motion (within stillness, motion). It is at such moments that we are able to receive the inspiration and guidance that characterize the Heaven realm.

    In Taoism we are all seen as manifestations of divine breath. When we connect to our larger vision, we inspire (draw in breath) and, in so doing, draw in a personal connection to the divine or the cosmos.

    The Principle of the Heaven triad is *Balance Brings Harmony.* As a personal interpretation of the Law, this Principle explores the meaning behind the symbol for the Tao (☯) , which illustrates the balance and interplay of yin and yang. We live in a culture that regards polarities as contradictory or adversarial, such as motion *or* stillness, doing *or* being. *Balance Brings Harmony* explores a different way to live with and enjoy (inJoy) the paradoxes intrinsic to our lives.

    The Practice of the Heavenly triad, *Embrace Wholeness (Tao),* draws from the *perspective* of the Law and sustains the *expression* of the Principle in your daily life. The exercises and meditations in this Practice provide you with the tools to move out of an *either/or* paradigm and ground you in specific and concrete ways as you move into a new relationship with dualities (and how to move beyond them) into the realm of thinking, feeling and being that is *all/and.*

CHAPTER 3

The Breath of Joy

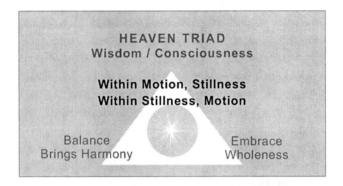

Within Motion, Stillness; Within Stillness, Motion
Law of the Heaven Triad

You must learn to be still in the midst of activity and to be
vibrantly alive in repose.
—Indira Gandhi

The first Law of the *Way of Joy*—*Within Motion, Stillness; Within Still-ness, Motion*—addresses the fundamental theme underlying the Heaven realm: How do we create a personal connection to an essence we might call Source, the universal consciousness that gives us inspiration and guidance?

Two of the American Heritage Dictionary definitions for 'inspire' are "to breathe" and "to breathe life into." Indeed, by focusing on your breath, you enter the state of consciousness where this Law of the Heaven triad can guide you to become centered in the midst of your full life.

In particular, it is through attention to your breath that you access what I call the "Observer Self," an internal aspect of ourselves that allows us to stand apart and witness our actions, our life. This Observer Self provides the link to the universal consciousness of the Heaven realm.

A Union of Opposites:

The stillness in stillness is not the true stillness; only when there is stillness in motion does the universal rhythm manifest.
—Old Taoist Text

Stillness in Motion is a common martial arts and Taiji principle that, in true Taoist fashion, creates a union of opposites. The Tao or yin/yang symbol, commonly characterized by a circle of dark within the light and a circle of light within the dark, acknowledges the relationship and interdependence of polarities. The concept of Stillness in Motion describes a state of being in which the practitioner strives to embody the eye of the storm, to find her or himself at a core center that is utterly still, relaxed, and present.

Yet at the heart of that deep internal stillness, motion continues. The heart continues to pump blood, the lungs continue to move air, the digestive system sorts and distributes energy and waste, the body is in a constant state of motion to sustain life. Similarly, the rock-quiet stillness of a mountain teems with movement—the activity of insects and animals, the roots stretching through dirt, around rocks, life growing and forming—even the wind in the trees can be part of the motion in stillness. At the Source of all-that-is, the quantum particles of our beings and of the world around us are in unending motion at the heart of stillness.

Because it is both so crucial and so difficult to achieve stillness in the midst of chaos, I'm devoting most of this chapter to the "Stillness in Motion" aspect of the Law, as compared to "Motion in Stillness." I believe that by focusing on how to achieve stillness, it will ultimately become clear how the stillness in motion and the motion in stillness happen simultaneously.

But There's No Time!

The idea of Stillness in Motion is particularly difficult for many of us in western culture to understand. First of all, it seems to me that we live in an era when we feel as if we have no time. The paradox of living in this age of technology is that time-saving devices appear to take away more time than they give. Our lives are so hectic that we end up panting even when we are not running. I've reminisced with old friends, remembering days when we might drop over at someone's house for a cup of tea. Now meeting for a cup of coffee near work often needs to be scheduled a month in advance. Time appears to be accelerating. How in the world will we ever catch up, much less achieve stillness?

Stillness in Motion: Externally, In the World Around Us

I remember complaining of this dilemma once in a master Chi Kung workshop I was taking with Dr. Quinn. "Everything is just moving too fast," I asserted, "I need to slow down!" Khaleghl cocked an eyebrow, grinned at me and said, "Maybe what you need to do is speed up!" I had a moment of feeling irritated by her remark and then relieved. I experienced the "joy slump" I mentioned previously when she spoke about the experience of acceleration when you are in an airplane taking off. As it increases speed, she pointed out, the pressure builds. Once the plane hits a certain altitude, however, there's a sense of being still. You don't have any sense of being in motion other than occasional shifts in air pressure or wind currents. If you can match your internal state of being with what is happening externally, she observed, it becomes a way to achieve stillness.

When I brought up Khaleghl's example in a discussion I was leading, one of my students, Lucinda, was reminded of body surfing. She said, "At first, it's all struggle, being thrashed about by the waves, but once you catch one it feels like you're not moving at all." She described "an incredible experience of stillness," followed by the realization that she was "absolutely flying towards the beach. It's an extraordinary experience," she concluded, "well worth being pummeled by many waves."

Another student, Reba, who is a black belt in Kajukenbo, said that when she is sparring, her focus is to empty her mind. To do this, she said she needed to apply the concept of stillness in motion. She said, "Being up against an opponent brings up issues of defensiveness, opposition, challenge and fear. Yet rather than try to think ahead, I need to empty my mind so that when something happens, I'm just there, present. I am totally whole and with the moment."

Jayne, another student of mine, told me about an extraordinary experience her grandmother used to tell her and her brother about when they were young. Jayne ultimately included the incident in a short story about her family and has given me permission to tell part of it here.

Jayne's grandmother, Belle, a young English woman living in Pontiac, Illinois, had been babysitting for some friends one day when a neighbor came by to warn her that a tornado was coming. Not having a storm cellar in her own home, Jayne's grandmother wrapped up the baby she was taking care of in a coat and left to find shelter at another neighbor's house a block and a half away. Her grandmother described a smell in the air that was like an electrical wire burning in dirt. Here is what Jayne writes in her grandmother's voice:

...I walked along, quick as I could, with my 'ead down.

Then I heard what sounded like a train coming through town. But I looked over at the tracks and there wasn't a train in sight. Then all of a sudden, the noise stopped and it got dead quiet. Quieter than church, even. No birds were a-singing, not one rustle of a leaf. Everything was so still...I never did see it...It snuck right up on me. I saw the sky turn from that strange green into a glowing blue. It was like the sun had come out but it was shining blue instead of yellow. That's when I felt myself get lifted up right off the ground and sucked up into a big gray tube...Well there was no time for me to get scared. I just held onto that baby for dear life and prayed God's will would save us both. Way up over my head were shining silver clouds, with white light flashing all around them. And spinning around the sides just above me were all sorts of things ...

...I tried not to (look down) because my feet were just dangling there, swaying this way and that. But when I did dare to look down, I saw rooftops going by. When I saw the flat, black-tarred roof of the cinder block factory where your Grandpa used to work, why I knew it had carried me all the way over Main Street to the other side of town.

...Well I kept my arms bundled tight around baby Sarah. ...When I was sure we were going to get sucked up...I'd feel something pulling us back down. Then I saw the lamp posts getting closer and prayed we weren't going to get dropped clear to the street. ...But then, like the Lord himself was reaching down and tugging on my overcoat, we would get lifted right back up toward the 'eavens. ...All of a sudden we just floated down towards the earth and were set down in a row of 'edges, gentle as could be. After I was able to get to my feet, I unwrapped my coat and there she was, little Sarah, still sound asleep.

When Jayne told me the story, she added that her grandmother remarked on "an eerie silence and eerie stillness" as she was being carried along. She assured me her grandmother didn't just invent stories like this. Jayne even did some research on tornados and said that even though her grandmother wouldn't have been picked up by anything as violent as a Class III tornado, she may have been pulled into a small funnel cloud. In her research Jayne found that descriptions of the inside of a funnel cloud were actually very similar to what her grandmother had experienced. Further corroborating her story was a man who actually witnessed Belle getting dropped into those shrubs. In fact, it became a town legend that 'Belle had gotten picked up by a tornado and Mr. So-and-so saw it happen!'

My own first experience of witnessing and thinking about Stillness in Motion was during my summer vacation between fourth and fifth grades. While playing at the seashore with my two younger brothers, I discovered that if I filled a sand pail with water and whirled around in a circle, I could swing the bucket out horizontally and not a drop of water would spill out.

When I described this experience to my science teacher at the beginning of the school year, she invited me to come to the seventh grade class and demonstrate my discovery. With a combination of trepidation and assertiveness, I marched into the circle of older girls and spun my pail in circles. The teacher subsequently engaged the class in a discussion of centrifugal force that I half-listened to, uncomprehending. What I did discover from that fifth grade experiment was that at the center of my spinning, the water in the pail appeared to have become totally still. This gave me, on a visceral level, the understanding of the concept that within motion lies stillness.

I believe that in order to sustain the acceleration of our speeded-up times, we absolutely need to cultivate our ability to be at the "eye of the storm." This doesn't mean to shut out chaos or acceleration around us, but to remain centered within it, like the water in that sand pail, while in relationship to it at the same time.

Stillness in Motion: Internally, In Our Own Lives

This idea of achieving a state of stillness in the middle of chaos is not just a principle useful to the martial artist, body surfer or pail slinger. It offers a life lesson that can be employed at times of overwhelm, conflict or stress. When there is so much going on around you that you feel like you don't know which end is up, or there is so much "brain mutter" going on in your mind that you forget even to breathe, you will not be operating at your full capacity or in relation to your internal guidance. Keeping an awareness of Stillness in Motion gives you the ability to stay calm and centered, relaxed and energized, even when you are actively engaged with what is happening around and within you.

A Moment of Stillness

To meet everything and everyone through stillness instead of mental noise is the greatest gift you can offer to the universe. I call it stillness, but it is a jewel with many facets: that stillness is also joy, and it is love.
—Eckhart Tolle

In the middle of his busy day, Manuel takes a moment to meditate. He sits and closes his eyes. As the events of the day continue to swirl around him, he slows down. He becomes quiet. From the silence, he moves into stillness. He focuses on the motion of his breath moving in and out. Within the momentum of a chaotic day, he has become still. (Within Motion, Stillness.) In the stillness of his meditation, he discovers his breath in motion. (Within Stillness, Motion.) Within the motion of his breath, his mind stops whirling, becomes still. (Within Motion, Stillness.) Within the stillness of his mind, his energy shifts, transforms. (Within Stillness, Motion.) When Manuel opens his eyes, the events in his workplace that had seemed overwhelming and unmanageable have a different quality. Everything seems to be going as it should.

Some people experience the kind of stillness Manuel achieved during his meditation as a visceral feeling, others hold it more as a mental awareness, while still others believe it is an attitude of consciousness. For me, stillness is all three, existing in both time and space as a state of suspension, a neutral zone where I can become close to the experience of divine influence, an entry into the state of being that Buddhists call mindfulness and, in essence, awake to the present moment or the presence of Now.

Time is not stopped, exactly, but it feels stretched out. Imagine lovers, focused only on each other, moving in slow motion during a candlelight dinner in a restaurant, alone in the crowded room. Referred to later as a "timeless" experience, the sensation is remembered forever. However, the experience of such timelessness does not require being in love. It can be experienced anytime. Perhaps in the middle of a city crowd at rush hour when, for no particular reason, you tune into the sound of an infant laughing, a coin dropping, or a particularly musical sneeze. Stillness exists in a rainstorm when you find yourself pausing for just a moment and doing nothing but listening to the rhythm of water dripping off a tree branch or onto the windowsill.

By entering the present moment in this way, you develop the ability to shift your experience of linear time. In a sense, we can enter a time out of time. Great spiritual masters, and now quantum physicists as well, teach us that time is not really linear. It is a construct that we as humans have put into place to make sense out of chaos. All time is simultaneous, and yet in the journey that we perceive from past to present to future there is a thread, a constancy, that we can discover. One constant we can depend on is that all things are in a state of change—motion.

To be in a state of stillness within that motion, or even chaos, brings us to a yin state of receptivity. It is a spacious state of being open to whatever might happen. Within stillness, you enter into a state of both inner and outer listening and in so doing, you become open to change, the inspiration and guidance of yang energy that characterize the Heaven Realm.

Even in moments of stress, contraction, or hopelessness, our experience can change almost instantly, as it did for Manuel. At times, when I've been preoccupied or anxious about issues that seemed very real and pressing, I've paused to breathe in the sound of the bubbling chortles of the creek near my house in Trinity County. The creek seems to cheer "Yippee! Yippee! Yippee!" From that stillness, something moves inside me, and I begin to hear my own core of merriment answering the call of the brook.

Of course, the more stressful things feel, the less likely we are to remember to breathe. Yet when you do take a moment simply to focus on nothing but the sound and sensation of breath moving in and out of your lungs, to literally listen to it, that action can change you and everything around you. Motivational speaker Wayne Dyer created the axiom, "Change the way you look at things, and the things you look at change." In his case, he's speaking about attitude and intention. What I'm speaking of here is the first step you can take to access and embody that intention: Just take a deep breath.

When we come to a place of centered breath, where breath is the only thing we're aware of, we can begin to *feel* our life force, a little bubble of joy. From there emerges the willingness, even eagerness, to go to the next breath and from there the willingness, delight even, to move on to the next moment.

So I'd like to ask you, as you read these words, *are you breathing?* Take a moment now (why not?) to focus on your breath. If you've been holding your breath, take a moment to sigh. Empty your lungs as fully as you can and then blow away any extra remaining breath in a few quick puffs. When you have exhaled completely, allow a full inhalation to come in. As you feel your lungs fill, see if you can experience nothing else, just the awareness of the air coming in.

The revered Vietnamese Buddhist master, Thich Nhat Hanh, teaches when you inhale, to think simply, "I am breathing in," when you exhale, think, "I am breathing out." He has said,

> Our true home is in the present moment.
> To live in the present moment is a miracle.
> The miracle is not to walk on water.
> The miracle is to walk on the green Earth
> in the present moment,
> to appreciate the peace and beauty

that are available now.
Peace is all around us—
in the world and in nature—
in our bodies and spirits.
Once we learn to touch this peace,
we will be healed and transformed.
It is not a matter of faith;
it is matter of practice.[1]

The Buddhist practice of being in the present moment begins with mindful conscious breath. In what might be seen as another paradox, there is a strong relationship between being in the present moment and being connected to Universal Source. Thus your breath is your entry to the Heaven realm. When you enter the paradox of Stillness in Motion, Motion in Stillness, you are then able to access that greater perspective of Heaven realm, to hold the whole, to connect to the larger Self.

Accessing the Observer Self

I saw my Lord with the eye of my heart and I said: Who art Thou? He said: Thou.
—Al-Halla

When we breathe into the present moment, we become one with what I call the "Observer Self" or what is also sometimes referred to in some spiritual or quantum scientific circles as the Witness. The Observer Self is the aspect of yourself that is separate from what is happening around you, from your reactions to any particular stimulus. It's the part of you able to simply look at what is happening around you or within you at any given moment without needing to react or change or engage. In its essence, the aspect that is the Observer Self is both detached and compassionate.

In the movie, *What the Bleep Do We Know?* physicist William Tiller claims we are all consciousness or spirit riding around in a body, what he humorously calls a "four-layer bio-body suit." Quantum physicists, as well as the great mystics, would have us look at this presence called the Observer. The Observer doesn't actually exist in any part of our body or brain. Rather it's an intangible aspect that exists in a state of stillness. Using all the senses you have available, your Observer picks up data, some 2,000 out of 40,000 stimuli that are around you. Your history governs to some degree what you notice, and your reactions depend on a myriad of causes. But the Observer Self, the one that is connected to the Heaven realm, to your inner sense of God or larger perspective, is neutral and everlasting.

When I was a little girl, I had a full-length mirror on my bedroom door. I used to stand in front of that mirror and block out all of my reflection except my eyes. Long before I had ever heard either the adage that the eyes are the window to the soul, I would gaze into my own eyes. I don't think I was motivated by vanity. Rather, I somehow knew instinctively there was something I was seeing there that was constant, unchanging. Now when I look at my reflection and let my vision widen, I can see that everything around my eyes has changed as I've aged, but there is still something I can see in my eyes that I saw as a five-year old.

Even though all of the cells of my body have died and new ones regenerated many times so that physically I am no longer made of the same matter, and even though over the course of my lifetime I have undergone many incarnations of the being I call my "self"—that is, the concept of who I am—there is one constancy. This presence or spirit has remained unchanging. It is the Observer Self, the thread that takes me through all the shifts and changes that have occurred in my evolution from that age to now.

Conclusion: How Stillness Saved My Life

I experienced the union of Stillness in Motion and Motion in Stillness in another more dramatic way in 1990. As I mentioned briefly in the previous chapter, I was hit by a car as I was walking across a street in San Francisco. Thrown up into the air by the impact, I felt as though my awareness had shrunk to a size that could fit on the head of a pin. This awareness was located right in the middle of my lower *tan tien* (also known by the Japanese word, *hara*) at the pit of my belly. I remember feeling surprised because in spite of my years doing martial arts, I somehow would have expected my consciousness to go to my upper *tan tien* (or sixth chakra, the third eye). I had the distinct image in that moment that my body was like a hull and my consciousness, my very essence or being, was a seed inside of that hull. Time suspended. As I floated in that suspension, I looked around at my inner silhouette with awe. I realized I had a choice. I could stay inside of this hull, my body, or I could leave. I felt no judgment, no despair, no fear, not even hope. I would say if I had any emotion at all, it was curiosity–what would I choose to do? At some point, I made an intentional decision to stay and opened my eyes. The pavement appeared to be coming up at me very fast. Instinctively, I tucked into an Aikido roll as I came down for a landing several car lengths from where I was hit.

Although I was thrown up in the air for only a fraction of a second, it was long enough for me to have a whole internal discussion. I experienced complete stillness as my body flew through the air and within that stillness I had a life-changing dialogue with myself. Within Motion, Stillness; Within Stillness, Motion.

Time stopped and my spirit, my larger Self, the Observer, was aware that I had a choice. It was not a given at that point in my life that I would choose to live. Even with the many privileges that I've had, I had experienced many periods when living seemed too painful, the world around me—personally and globally—seemed too out of balance, or simply wrong. But at that moment of stillness, hovering between life and death, I had a clear sense I was being called to embrace life in a renewed and different way.

In that one moment, I had a visceral sense of being a consciousness living inside of a container. Normally that consciousness feels pervasive, living in every cell of my body, whether I am aware of it or not. At that moment of near death, however, I felt a contraction, a concentration pinpointing into one small area, as an aspect of myself readied itself to undergo a profound transformation.

That moment out of time reminds me of the assertion from quantum physics that any particle—whether it be an atom within a molecule or a proton within an atom—is actually, as University of Oregon physics Professor Dr. Amit Goswami says, "a cloud of possibility." During that endless moment of being suspended between staying in my body and leaving, between living and dying, that pinpoint of awareness, my consciousness—"I"—became simply a cloud of possibility. Within that cloud, I opened to the information that I needed to live a different way, to stop trying to fit myself into any form other than that directed by my own spirit.

To experience stillness in your life does not require shutting down your senses or building a barrier to the chaos of an energetic, alive and unpredictable world. Through the power of your breath and attention, you can sustain an awareness of that inner space of quiet constancy, the peaceful Observer, while the world around you spins and twirls. At the same time, when we take a moment, even in the midst of chaos, to stop and breathe, opening the door to our Observer Self, we gain insights, making the kind of internal movement that can change our lives in profound ways. Each breath brings us to the present moment that opens us to inspiration from the Heaven Realm—the inspiration that, in turn, ignites our joy.

CHAPTER 4
The Dance of Joy

```
        HEAVEN TRIAD
     Wisdom / Consciousness

      Within Motion, Stillness
      Within Stillness, Motion

   Balance                    Embrace
   Brings Harmony             Wholeness
```

Balance Brings Harmony
Principle of the Heaven Triad

Harmony and well-being are born from balancing extremes.
—Ma Deva Padma

The Principle (Human realm) interprets and applies the information of its corresponding Law (Heaven realm) in ways that are personal and unique to each individual. As the Principle of the Heaven triad, *Balance Brings Harmony* explores how the perspective and inspiration of the Law *Within Stillness, Motion; Within Motion, Stillness,* might be used in our own lives. This Principle of examines how to live with the co-existence of opposites. In fact, it is the delicate back-and-forth that, in the apparent paradox between stillness and motion, allows Harmony.

Opposites Polarized
In Western culture we are taught that opposites, by their very nature, are polarized and compete for dominance. One excludes the other. Blocking our ability to find the harmony between paradoxical elements, I believe this perspective permeates every aspect of our lives. When we don't see the harmony possible in opposites, we create a culture of dominance and submission, of right and wrong, where for someone to win, another

has to lose. Take, as a common example, an issue such as land use that splits community members into factions. One side's sure only the ecologist is "right"; the other side, the developer. As each side intensifies its assertion, communication often becomes increasingly polarized, leading to divisiveness and struggle for dominance.

I also think this "right-wrong" polarization invades our inner landscape, our thought processes, our own personal choices. For example, you might have an inner argument about whether you should eat an ice cream cone. One voice might say, "No, you wanted to get healthier and more fit. Eating ice cream would sabotage your commitment to a low-fat diet!" The other voice might argue, "But you deserve some sweetness. It's been a such a hard day, you should indulge yourself." The two voices go to war with one another, struggling for dominance. For many of us, this kind of inner conflict happens many times every day, whether it is deciding whether or not to finish a mystery or get a full night's sleep, take time to go Salsa dancing or be a responsible parent and stay home to help with the art project, enjoy learning something new or give up because you feel overwhelmed and don't "get it," and so on.

The concept of harmony can shed a different light on the relationship between different elements, even those that are polarized. The dictionary defines "harmony" as a musical agreement of sounds or tones, a pleasing arrangement of parts. Harmony, it's important to observe, is not unison. The two or more notes that are played together differ from one another, might even be called "opposite" in some way, like high notes and low notes. Together these differing tones create a rich and multi-layered texture that is harmony. It is the bringing together and balancing of these diverse voices that forms "a chord," or accord. Interestingly, a second definition of harmony refers to "accord," together with "internal calm."

Assessing Balance

To apply the Principle of *Balance Brings Harmony* to your life, you can begin by asking about your own interpretation of harmonizing stillness and motion:

- How can you balance the acts of giving and receiving? Of expanding energy to get things done and contracting energy for rest?

- How can you experience harmony within your own psyche, and so create internal peace? How can you create balance in the external world—your community and environment—and be in harmony with your surroundings?

- How might you live in balance in all levels of awareness—physical, emotional, mental, and spiritual—where all of the "notes" of your internal voices and external expressions are included?

The Balanced Harmony of Tao

One of the primary Taoist teachings holds that opposites are, in fact, complementary and interdependent. Two sides, yin and yang, are in constant play, balancing one another in a state of harmonious co-existence symbolized by the Tao pictogram. ☯ In the world of Chi Kung, where human beings are conduits between heaven/inspiration (yang/creative) and earth/creation (yin/receptive), balance can be found by drawing Heaven down to Earth and Earth up to Heaven. Bringing Heaven to Earth happens any time you succeed in making a dream or vision manifest. Drawing Earth up to Heaven might be experienced at times you feel stuck by taking a moment to stop grappling with the problem and instead look at the whole picture. Doing this, you surrender and open to your inner guidance for inspiration and discover how to regain your flow.

Balancing Conflicting Elements of Our Experience

Help us to be the always hopeful gardener of the spirit who knows that without darkness nothing comes to birth as without light nothing flowers.
—May Sarton

When we choose to move out of the polarized opposites of the right/wrong paradigm, we enter a whole new world of harmonic possibilities, where we live in the balance between Heaven and Earth. In her beautifully illustrated divinatory card set, "Tao Oracle: An Illustrated New Approach to the I Ching," Ma Deva Padma offers her interpretation of the hexagram for Conflict: "When an individual or group feels strongly about an idea, a proposal or a certain way of doing things, it is easy to lose sight of a bigger picture, where each vantage point offers a unique and valuable perspective. And when opposing sides of a conflict get 'locked in' to their positions, both lose the perspective that is needed to come to resolution."[1]

On a community level, I believe the movement to explore new forms of mediation, conflict resolution and cultural competency has taken huge strides. One example is Sharon Ellison's brilliant work on *Powerful Non-Defensive Communication*™, a new model of communication that has the power to diffuse defensiveness and power struggle.[2] Another example of historic proportions is Desmond Tutu's Truth and Reconciliation Commission in South Africa, a process through which the kind of severely polarized positions resulting from oppression and war were processed in innovative ways. There are countless other examples of new ways we are learning how to resolve polarized differences.

As for inner conflict, what does it mean to be a balanced individual when as humans we exist in a sea of complex, often conflicting, thoughts and feelings? To be balanced, I think, a person needs to maintain an overview, access the inner stillness of the Observer in order to cultivate a detached compassion for one's own inner world. I believe we have the ability to train ourselves to listen to and honor the different voices that war inside of our psyches.

For example, what if you train yourself to hear the voice insisting on an ice cream cone as a yearning for sweetness and enjoyment rather than as a saboteur, an enemy to struggle against, where fun is pitted against health? If you explore new ways for the part of you that wants to eat more mindfully to work with the part that wants to be comforted or sweetened, you might discover what underlies the yearning. You might then satisfy it while avoiding the "sugar blues," that crash that comes after the "sugar high" binge. To balance sweetness (or comfort or reward) with health habits could become a whole new experiment where neither side wins or loses.

Does that mean you have to always be austerely "healthy" and never eat anything that is not perfectly nourishing? I don't think so.

Balance is an evolutionary process. There's no set script as we seek it. You might succeed in having one scoop of ice cream or look for alternatives with a different kind of sweetener than sugar. You may sometimes decide to call a friend and have a good talk instead of running to the store for a treat. You may find you can let yourself feel the freedom of the occasional splurge and still make meaningful progress toward your health goals. You may also learn to cultivate new "treats" that nurture both your immediate need for freedom or comfort and your spirit/body health.

When you can view diverse stances as enriching rather than problematic, you'll give birth to the expression of your true nature, which, I believe, is powerfully harmonious. Here you become able to hold more than one "note" at a time in a pleasing and enhancing way. This, in turn, ripples out to create harmony in larger and larger circles. As Padma says, "Both energy and vision are contagious, whether the contagion is defensiveness, anger and fear, or the understanding that each of us is a unique and treasured member of a greater whole. What kind of contagion we spread is a choice that is available to us, all of the time."[3] If we cultivate our ability to see ourselves and everyone else as essential and valuable to the whole, we can indeed become the transporters of inner and outer peace.

Harmony may be found in the balance between giving and receiving, birthing and dying, loving and receiving love, creating and releasing, expanding and contracting, opening and closing. You may give a special gift and feel fulfilled by receiving a friend's deep appreciation. You may be holding the person you are in love with and feel immeasurable bliss and simultaneously feel the pain of what it would be like to lose her or him.

We can certainly feel joy without consciously feeling sorrow, or sorrow without joy. At the same time, when you allow yourself to move between one aspect and the other, to experience both sorrow and pleasure, for example, as interconnected, even simultaneous, you enter what has been called the "dewy-eyed state"[4] where there is joy in your heart at the same time as there are tears in your eyes. To be in balance is to embrace the whole of your experience. This practice is, at its essence, at the heart of the Tao.

Journal Entry: As I walked out the door, I could smell the damp – unusual here for the hot dry fiery season of summer. As I walk through the woods, I can hear distant thunder and see the sky darkening. Later as I do my Chi Kung and meditation practice by the creek, there is a downpour although the sun is still bright overhead. Perfect Tao moment.

Balancing Cycles of Expansion and Contraction

Living in Luna…taught me that one of the best ways to find balance is to go to extremes.
—Julia Butterfly Hill

For many years in my life as an actor and performer, I found myself repeating a cycle again and again. I would create and perform a show, feel exhilarated with the process and with my achievement. Whether the material was developed as a solo or with my theater company, I loved the rush of inspiration, the drive to express myself. I felt empowered, motivated, and strong, in love with the process of creation, with the experience of sharing with an audience, the deep sense of connection to Source.

When the run of the show ended, I would crash. Exhausted after a large exertion, I was always certain I'd reached the end of my creative potential. I had shot my wad, given it all I could, and had nothing left to say. The rest of my life looked bleak. Harshly dismissive of my creative work, in fact of my whole creative being, I would go over everything I had done in the show that I didn't like. Regardless of reviews, of how the piece had been received, of who liked it and who didn't, I would focus almost exclusively on the negative and the critical. The underlying message to myself was "Who do you think you are? You have nothing worth saying. Get back into that box where you belong. Don't get too big or too visible."

Once "back in the box," I became stagnant. My Spirit felt inert, my creativity numb. After a period of depression and despair, I would eventually kick myself into gear and rev up for the next show. I'd go through some doubt and anxiety in the early raw stages of the creation process, then become inspired and begin to enjoy myself again. I would create and perform the piece, feel whatever success I experienced, and, once it was over, crash once more.

After many years of repeating this cycle, I began to think of it as an addictive pattern I wanted to change. In a nutshell, I recognized that every time I threw myself into the frenzy of putting on a production to stave off feelings of depression, I was forcing myself back onto the same old treadmill. I decided to quit performing and didn't return to the stage for ten years. During that hiatus, by detaching from any situation where my ego would be defined by how I saw my "worth" as a theater artist, I could see the pattern I had been experiencing in my creative work: expand—contract—expand—contract—expand—contract.

At the peak of my expression, when I felt expansive and open, I was relaxed, accepting, and connected. My experience was one of allowing creativity to be expressed through me, where my impulse and my joy were unwavering. When I contracted, I felt disconnected from inspiration, the perspective of the Heaven realm.

I've observed that other people also seem to experience times of wilting, of self-doubt or discouragement, a kind of post-partum depression after achieving a particular goal. Whether it be writing a thesis, winning a challenging argument, moving to a new place, or anything else that takes a concentrated or creative effort to manifest, of bringing Heaven down to Earth, the time of expansion is likely to be followed by a time of contraction. How we achieve the balance between cycles of expansion and contraction is vital to our harmony, and I believe we've been given a lot of cultural messages that damage our capacity to create this balance.

The Socio-Economic World versus The Natural World

In my social studies class in high school, I remember learning that, in order to thrive under capitalism, companies need to be in an ever-expanding state of economic growth. We in the United States live in a political and social climate where contraction (or a time of non-productivity) is considered to be a malfunction. This paradigm trickles down into our consciousness and impacts our daily lives and the choices we make.

Capitalism has traditionally held that expansion is good and contraction is bad, to be minimized and overcome as rapidly as possible. Growth is required, and growth occurs only through expansion. On an individual level, if someone succeeds at achieving a goal, there is then pressure to focus on the next goal. There may be some allowance for a short vacation, but the question soon arises—"What next?"

I believe this perspective creates an unrelenting pressure and lies at the root of the disease of "just one more thing-itis," which drives many of us into the kind of stressful, unsatisfying multi-tasking that in turn contributes to the experience of accelerated time referred to in the previous chapter. "Down time" or rest is, at best, necessary but to be dispensed with as efficiently and invisibly as possible. I'm often struck by how many students and friends have said they feel ashamed to admit they have taken time during the day to read a novel, do a crossword puzzle, or take a nap. Even vacation time, for most people, is barely long enough to stop the internal buzz before picking up their "real life" once again. What matters is production—what you do, not who you are, never mind how you "be."[5]

In contrast, in Nature expansion and contraction are inherent cycles. To polarize aspects of these cycles as "good" or "bad" requires a separation from the world around us—a world where blossoms open to the sun and close at dusk, where the ocean swells and recedes with the tides, where day turns to night which then turns to day, where our very breath and pulse depend on the constancy of the expansion and contraction of our lungs and our hearts.

The natural world teaches us there is a time to open, a time to close, a time to be at full peak, a time to lie fallow. I can think of no expansion on this planet of living beings that is not followed, in some way, by contraction, which in turn is followed by expansion, then by contraction. The pattern is simply part of being in a living, breathing world.

As I mused on this natural cycle, I finally had to ask myself, "If you're going to contract anyway, do you want to go down kicking and screaming, or do you want to find another way?" This brought more questions:

• How might I embrace contraction in a way that would be restful and self-nurturing instead of stifling and self-punishing?

• If I could anticipate and embrace the time of contraction with an intention to remain at peace, how would I prepare for it?

• What would contraction feel like if it were simply the other side of expansion, if I looked at it as a balance between yin and yang, being and doing, drawing in and sending out?

- Might I be able to experience the state of being, of listening, of allowing, to be as instructive and valuable as doing, expressing, and producing?

I invite you to consider your own answers to these questions.

The Yang of Expansion, The Yin of Contraction

On the most fundamental level, expansion radiates energy out, as with an activity, a project, some form of self-expression. It is, in its nature, yang. Contraction draws energy in, as in the state of receptivity, replenishing, drifting, or simply being. It is, in its nature, yin. Yang correlates to light, to emergence. Yin correlates to darkness, to withdrawal. Each is a vital part of our life cycle.

I believe that we expand and contract in small, subtle ways every day. One obvious example is to have a good night's sleep after a full, productive day. Here there is ease in contracting, knowing you can relax and have a period of restoration before the demands of the next day. Yin leads to yang, which, in turn, leads back to yin. And it's in the fine balance between yin and yang that we find ourselves in harmony with the world around us, a state of being that allows Joy to flow.

Balance = yin —> yang —> yin —> yang —> yin —> yang

When the cycles of contraction and expansion, yin and yang, are out of balance, we suffer, become dysfunctional, and find ourselves out of harmony with the world around us. When you have been in a yin state for too long, you will tend to feel uninspired and lethargic. For instance, have you ever experienced sleeping for too long, perhaps taken a nap during the day, only to find yourself feeling waterlogged and fuzzy-brained for the rest of the day?

On the other hand, at the completion of some major endeavor, have you ever found yourself in the kind of state I described after I had completed a theater production? Simply put, if you spend too much time putting energy out, you become depleted—a more common complaint for most people. Have you ever experienced being under pressure for a sustained period of time to complete a project at work, or to plan a big event like a party or a wedding? You promise yourself that just as soon as it is over, you will take a break, take some time to recuperate, do something good for yourself. When that time finally comes and you are ready to relax, you get sick and you spend your time "off" with nose drops and cough syrup. One of my students, a college professor, told me she experienced this one spring break after another during her career.

Journal entry: I've been noticing lately that when I talk to people at times when I crave solitude, am tired, or in another kind of contraction, I invariably want to eat something sweet or over-eat. I have realized that, in fact, I am actually trying to bring energy back in to replenish myself after putting too much energy out.

Yin and Yang: A Dance of Balance

In the I Ching, yin, the state of receptivity, relates to Earth. Yang, the bringer of change, relates to Heaven, which includes sun, rain, astronomical and astrological influences, the movement of the planets and cosmic bodies. These Heavenly yang forces effect powerful change on the Earthly yin, which receives the influence of yang (Heaven), then returns again to its natural state of receptivity. So while yang is transformative and powerful, it is short-lived and easily spent. Yin is the more constant, tranquil state. In this context, the earth we live on remains in a state of receptivity, influenced and changed by the heavenly influences, and returning once again to receptivity.

The flow between yang and yin is like a dance. Just as when you dance with someone who moves backward as you step forward and vice versa, you can learn to dance with your cycles of yin and yang. In the different styles of Taiji or other walking Chi Kung forms, which are sometimes compared to dance, the practitioner learns to play with this balancing act in different ways. In solo practice, she or he strives to create an internal experience of balance on a physical plane, mindfully shifting weight back and forth between the left and right feet as the form progresses. This physical experience of balance contributes to balance on an emotional level, as the mind quiets and the spirit plays, creating the calm equilibrium of meditation.

In the Tai Chi practice called "push hands," as well as in a form of Ba Gua taught to me by Taiji Master Dr. Franklin Kwong, the point of connection between two practitioners becomes another area in which to explore balance. Here you focus both on your own internal balance and on the point of balance in the connection between the two of you. In both push hands and in the solo forms, Tai Chi practitioners learn to move into a field of harmony within themselves and with their surroundings.

If you think of yourself as playing at push hands, being a co-creator with Universal Source in the dance of your life, you will find you can enjoy the give and take, the balance of yin and yang in that creative process.

When you allow yourself to follow energy as it swells and ebbs in a natural flow, and you become intentional about how to respond to that flow, you will find that, in the end, you will enjoy the very act of balancing itself as it takes you deeper—via a labyrinth rather than a straight line—to your own connection to and expression of that Source.

The Yin of Yang, and the Yang of Yin

The constant cycle of yin and yang, of receiving and giving, creates a loop of reciprocity. At the same time, each contains its opposite within itself as is depicted in the pictogram of yin and yang that symbolizes the Tao. ☯ Remember, you can see a point of light inside the dark and one of dark inside the light. Yin exists inside of yang, and yang lives inside of yin. Thus it is important we recognize that at the heart of contraction lives expansion, and that expansion contains, at its core, contraction.

On the most fundamental physical level of our breath, exhalation correlates to expansion, which is outgoing, sending—yang. In fact, people often use an out breath to accompany an effort, such as lifting a heavy garbage bag or pushing when birthing in labor. Inhalation correlates to contraction, which is incoming, receiving—yin. When you want to calm yourself or slow down, you may tell yourself to "take a deep breath." To be even more literal, when you exhale, you send energy out, which feeds the plants in the form of carbon dioxide. When you inhale, you draw energy in from plants as oxygen. This cycle of giving and receiving is one of the basic ways that we live in reciprocal, harmonious balance with the natural world around us.

At the same time, at the heart of the expansion and contraction of our breath you will find its opposite, just as in the Tao symbol. When you inhale to draw in air (yin), you actually expand your lungs (yang). This opens up internal space, creates an *internal* expansion. Similarly, during the labor of childbirth, it is the contractions that provide an internal opening, an internal expansion of the uterus and pelvic bones to make space for the baby's passage from womb to air. This is the yang inside of the yin.

Conversely, when you exhale, your lungs contract. This is what sends the breath out. The internal compression that allows for the release of breath is like a bellows feeding a flame. Think of times when you are "in the zone," getting things done, in your creative element, when you've experienced an internal sense of relaxation, of release, even as you are in the middle of highly focused work. This is the yin inside of the yang.

I find that this understanding of yin inside of yang, yang inside of yin is useful when applied to any kind of stretching, whether physically, emotionally, or mentally. For example, I have noticed when I feel emotionally off-balance, I usually also feel tight somewhere in my body and my mind. When I stretch and practice Chi Kung, I believe I both literally and metaphorically balance the right and left (yang and yin) hemispheres of my brain, and in so doing create well-being on all levels.

It's vital to breathe as you stretch. In most kinds of stretching, whether in dance, martial arts, yoga, athletics or other types of exercise, if you hold your breath, you are likely to limit or even block any expansion of your muscles. At the same time, if you use your breath to find the yin (release) inside of the yang (expanse), the stretch will not only go further, it will also feel more pleasurable. You can drop into a relaxed, restful state as you exhale your breath out instead of tightening up as your lungs contract. I've also experimented in my own stretch practice by placing myself into a particular posture and breathing in. I imagine my muscles expanding, widening, becoming plumper as I inhale. That is the yang/expansion inside of the yin/inhalation. Then, when I exhale (yang), I release that "plumpness," which allows my muscles to stretch a little further and allows for the flow of chi. This is the yin (release) inside of the yang (exhalation).

If we take this premise of yin at the heart of yang, yang at the heart of yin as a premise for life's expansions and contractions, then it follows that we must be able to open internally to the experience of life's contractions if we are to become balanced. When you are internally receptive (you expand inside to take in the change), you no longer need to fight the experience of going into your contracted smaller self. Just as your lungs expand when you breathe in, you can internally expand to contractions that happen in your life, moving with grace into a state of "being-ness" instead of "doing-ness."

Balance of Three

Chi Kung Master Quinn has said that our energy can be divided into three parts. In order to be in balance, one third of our energy needs to be expressed, go out, for example, in service to others, which is yang. One third needs to come in as replenishment, which is yin. She describes the final third as "energy going into the bank," into our reserve, which might also be seen as yin. Here, the balance between yin and yang becomes a balance among three aspects.

I'll never forget the exhilaration of my first rafting experience on the Trinity River. Much of the trip involved lazily floating down the river, drinking in the cool fresh air, paddles resting on the sides of the raft as our guide, Jigmae, pointed out an eagle nest here, signs of a bear there. Only when we got to the rapids did we become very active, for it would not do to continue to drift indolently into the white water and get tossed like a cork. Nor did it make sense to paddle furiously in a current that effortlessly carried us forward anyway. It interested me to note that the focused times of paddling the rapids themselves were much fewer than the times of being carried by the current, and to see that even when we were totally relaxed, putting out no effort, we were still carried forward by the flow of the river. It reminded me of Khaleghl's concept of two-thirds replenishment to one-third expression. The message I got from this excursion was "There is a time to drift, a time to paddle"—a useful metaphor in my life when I forget I am not meant to just "do, do, do."

Masaro Emoto, the Japanese scientist who has done such groundbreaking work with the study of *Hado* (the vibration) of water, has also speculated about the concept of a three-part balance based on yin and yang. He has said:

> We know that water is described as H_2O. If we were to look at love and gratitude as a pair, gratitude is the H and love is the O. Water is the basis that not only supports but also allows the existence of life. In my understanding of the concept of yin and yang, in the same way there is one O and two Hs, we also need one part yang/love to two parts yin/gratitude, in order to come to a place of balance in the equation.[6]

I believe that many people actually live out the reverse of this interpretation of balance. People tend to place two thirds of their energy on doing (yang) and one third (if that much) on non-doing or being (yin). I also believe that this is a socially expected norm. Given the values of this post-industrial culture, times of just "being," of lying fallow, in the way of the earth after a rainstorm, can be a very difficult to accept, let alone embrace.

Resisting Yin

If you are someone who does not take enough time to rest because of life's demands, or you tend to be a "Type A" personality, a time of non-doing can be frustrating and may even appear to prevent you from doing what you want to do. By its very nature, non-productive contraction can appear in many guises—you may feel stuck in a rut or find that what worked to get you going in the past no longer does.

Contraction often occurs at times when it is the very opposite of what you think you need, when you have a deadline to meet or obligations to fulfill, when you are craving momentum or inspiration. In fact, in a world of "do-ers" based on economic necessity and cultural expectations, just "being"—whether due to a layoff, a disability, or simply feeling drained—is one major cause for depression.

Contraction can frequently make you feel small and insignificant. It might also take the shape of a "wince memory"—something from your recent or distant past that makes you cringe when you think of it. For instance, have you ever experienced a situation where you took a risk and said or did something, and then became concerned it was inappropriate and spent hours or days afterwards kicking yourself for being so stupid? In taking the risk, you expanded your energy field. Then, not making room for or expecting contraction, you might have found that fear or shame took over, pushing you back into smallness. That feeling of shame might or might not be appropriate, but it becomes a way in which you feel reduced.

When blame or shame is part of the contraction, people tend to either push through the contraction and become more aggressive (the insecure egotist), or they succumb to it, experience themselves as diminished and exhibit low self-esteem.

In any of these cases, contraction can be frightening or demoralizing. Response to contraction can also appear as defiance or apathy, as in someone who says, "Who cares? I can't make a difference anyway, so I may as well just not try."

Accessing Joy in Contraction

My observations about cycles of expansion and contraction led me to an inquiry that continues to this day: How do we experience both expansion and contraction in a way that is balanced? Part of the answer, of course, is to accept our contraction as a healthy part of the cycle of growth. Then we can sink into the contraction and rest, thereby nurturing the seeds for the next expansion.

I believe the cultivation of emotional balance is critical for people who are committed to their own healing path. I think this balance comes from the ability to allow a wide range of emotions and thoughts to flow through you while not being so overtaken by one emotion that you lose your awareness of the bigger picture.

When we are out of balance, we either feel overwhelmed and chaotic or numb and shut down. We experience feelings like rage, depression (rage turned inward), and despair. Some people try to push these feelings away and focus only on the positive in a search of inner peace. While I agree with many of the ideas behind theories like the Law of Attraction and the Power of Positive Thinking—that how we live energetically attracts more of the same—I also believe it is critical to embrace the totality of who we are.

Harmony, remember, comes from the balance of several notes occurring at the same time to create a chord. Energetically, this means experiencing several different vibrations at the same time. On an emotional level, to feel *accord* requires us to cultivate the ability to not forget one aspect of self in the experience of another aspect of self.

This means *not* to try to rise above less desirable emotions, so-called "negative" feelings. It means to have compassion, patience and respect for any inner voice clamoring to be heard. I believe that every aspect of self has value.

If, as we have seen, at the core of yin (contraction) lies yang (expansion), then when you are feeling small or tight, shut down, it follows that this would be a time to cultivate an *internal* expansion. That internal opening leads to surrender—a form of acceptance, not defeat. Given that this moment of your cycle will come one way or another, see if you can find ways to embrace it before you find yourself inevitably collapsing into it. During this time you cannot produce. All you can "do" is "be." What would happen if you assume the contraction is not the enemy, but is rather leading you where you need to go?

Asking yourself to accept a contraction, to drop into it and go where it takes you, instead of pushing to do more, requires a great deal of trust. It is a big demand when you are not flowing easily, when you are dealing with resistance either internally or because of external circumstances. However, when you truly surrender to contraction—as opposed to *trying* to surrender, which implies a built-in resistance—you will discover unlimited resources of information and replenishment.

This is the time to open to your innermost thoughts, even if it means hearing voices you would prefer to keep silent. These thoughts are angels of information. They may sometimes appear to be condemning judges who label your limitations as bad, bringing with them feelings of hopelessness. Such feelings usually arise because the angels are trying to get your attention. The more you ignore them, the more they are apt to become increasingly loud and hostile, usually in the voices of old authorities or parent figures. However, if you listen for the gold inside of the harangue, you will often find a fierce protector who needs a new job description.

My partner Sherry once told me that during a time when she was being tormented by a harsh "inner critic" who shamed her, mocking her efforts and ridiculing her dreams, she decided to dialogue with this voice. She learned that the voice was, in fact, trying to prevent her from being hurt or disappointed. Telling it she was no longer willing to listen to demeaning or minimizing messages, she asked the voice to become a "Quality Control Expert," whose task would be to encourage her with suggestions about how to succeed. Through this internal opening, she was released from the pain of contraction.

Contraction requires letting go—letting go of all external concerns, going back to the core, letting in whatever needs to be there so you can ultimately be in restfulness, acceptance, forgiveness, inner peace. This isn't so you can become a "better" person or because you should be more "spiritual." Rather, by allowing the natural course of internal expansion to take place and thereby aligning with the natural flow between contraction and expansion, you can eliminate suffering and learn what can be learned *only* in that stage of the cycle.

In the case of my pattern of post-show contraction, it was only when I began to recognize that contraction is not only an inevitable part of an ongoing cycle, but also that *it actually creates inner expansion,* that I could begin to enjoy my post-performance spell. And when I relaxed and opened inside of my contraction, I discovered I was able to observe my own fears and judgments dispassionately instead of battering myself down with them. These thoughts have included honest and constructive evaluations of what I like about any given performance and what I wish to improve. I have found when I balance my intention to listen deeply with letting go of controlling any outcome, I can receive and appreciate whatever lessons my "quality control experts" bring me. In so doing, I move into a state of true replenishment.

If, when you enter a time of non-doing, you can intentionally shift your focus to sorting, listening and replenishing, you will find yourself able to enter a time of contraction mindfully and with anticipation of the rejuvenation it offers. In this way you will be able not only to make peace with the inevitability of contraction, but even to honor it. If the productive aspect of you protests, you can confidently assure it you will be able to accomplish even more when you return to your yang state.

Rest in Work: The Yin Inside of Yang

Just as you can find an internal expansion inside of contraction, outer expansion holds contraction at its core. When you express yourself or create, you create form out of chaos. It is the shaping of formlessness (yin) that becomes the expression, the emergence of form (yang). And I believe it's when we relax inside of an expansion that we best allow our creative or expressive impulse to take shape.

The renowned Jungian story-teller Clarissa Pinkola Estes relates a tale about the famed Picasso. One day, Picasso was standing in his garden, looking at the colors and textures around him. His neighbor came by, leaned on the fence, and said, "Pablo, hello—looks like you are resting today, good for you." Picasso responded by saying, "No, today I'm working." The next day, Picasso had set up an easel and was painting furiously, clearly consumed with putting colors on the canvas. His neighbor again leaned on the fence and said, "Ah, Pablo, today you are working," to which Picasso replied, "No, today I am resting."

In a culture where you are defined by what you do, and where what you do is "a result of your efforts," it seems contradictory to think of production or expansion as release or letting go, of effortlessly allowing your energy to come forth and radiate. The release and relaxation at the core center of the expansion of your energy field is the yin at the core of the yang.

In the case of Picasso, what felt like "work" was the time of his contraction, which contained an inner expansion—in other words, it was the yang expansion inside of the yin contraction, the "doing" inside of his state of "being." His "rest" was the time when he released and allowed energy to come through him (yin), giving it shape and form (yang), It was the yin inside of the yang, the "just being" at the core of his "doing."

This concept of yin at the center of yang, and yang at the center of yin is the way we manifest the Heaven Law of this triad, *Within Motion, Stillness; Within Stillness, Motion.* We are achieving balance by holding all that is in our lives as integrated rather than in conflict. In the next section, we'll look at how the ego plays a role in our ability to ultimately achieve harmony, within ourselves, within our community, and with the Heaven realm, our source of inspiration.

Balancing the Ego and the Greater Self: A Link to the Heaven Realm

The ego holds our sense of individuality, helping us function in a world of illusion where we experience ourselves as matter.
—Sherry Mouser

In the second chapter of this book, I said that in the Heaven realm we are all part of a great Cosmic gem—the we-are-all-one consciousness.

It's in the Human realm, we each express a unique facet of that gem, and I believe the ego is a tool for that individual expression.

The way I see it, ego is what makes you recognizable as you and me recognizable as me. And while ego is only temporal, I believe it is capable of great transformation and can play an important part in both spiritual evolution and expression.

Sadly, I believe that all too often in meditative and spiritual practices, ego gets a bad rap. For many people, the concept of ego has come to mean an aspect of self that we need to constantly guard against, to overcome or transcend. It has become synonymous with false pride, a sense of superiority or attachment to the illusions of the material world, particularly through our perceptions or personality. It has become the irreconcilable polar opposite of our "higher self," threatening to throw us off our spiritual and/or ethical path.

This attitude is so pervasive we almost adopt it by osmosis. I experienced this even as a child. I grew up in a musical family, where every child learned to play the piano. Sometimes when I was practicing, I would just stop, sit on the piano bench, and daydream about being famous.

My father was well known in his field at the time, so fame did not hold any particular illusion for me as guaranteeing happiness or a better life. Even as a kid, I think I was well aware of the pitfalls and the demands that fame brought. For me being famous was not so much about being on an ego trip as experiencing a sense of wanting to tap into my own wisdom and connect with others. When I fantasized about being interviewed on the Johnny Carson Show, I imagined being able to give a gift from my heart to people, to millions of people. What I was picturing in my child mind was how many hearts I could reach and how soon with the message I carried inside me about love and joy.

For years after, I felt some shame about that memory because it seemed so egotistical. "Oh yeah, don't do any of the hard work or discipline. Just daydream yourself as being more important than you really are." I now believe, however, those childish daydreams were an inspiration for the person I felt I'd love to be—someone who could deliver a message that would help people love themselves and one another. Whether I were to achieve that dream in the way in which I fantasized it or not is not what is important here. I believe what is relevant about any youthful fantasy is what we do with that early impulse. How do we balance those immature ego impulses with guidance from the Higher Self?

I have come to believe ego has its rightful place as a part of my spiritual practice. I believe it can contribute to an experience of greater consciousness, of connection to Spirit instead of being an aspect that separates us from Source. Modern dance pioneer Martha Graham said in this oft-quoted statement:

> There is a vitality, a life force, a quickening that is translated through you into action. And because there is only one of you in all time, this expression is unique. And if you block it, it will never exist through any medium and will be lost. The world will not have it. It is not your business to determine how good it is, nor how valuable it is, nor how it compares with other expressions. It is your business to keep it yours clearly and directly.

The Pitfalls of Ego

Zen Master Genpo Roshi has described ego as being nothing more than a concept. Imagine how often people change the "concept" of who they think they are over the course of a lifetime. At any given time, we define ourselves—who we are and how we function in the world—through our ego. Yet I do think there are some risks involved in how the ego functions, both in terms of being over-inflated and in terms of being weak or underdeveloped. Sometimes I think of the inflated ego as simply a child of our Greater Self, who can express Spirit in a myriad of ways. However, in its naiveté or innocence, ego often believes it is Destiny, the purveyor of the Whole Picture, of Reality. This, to me, is where ego can become a carrier of self-deception and illusion. In reference to *The Divine Romance* by Paramahansa Yogananda, Brother Anandamoy has said, "Beneath the wave of our consciousness is the infinite ocean of (God's) consciousness. The wave forgets it is part of the ocean…it has become isolated from oceanic power."[7] The ego, or the personality, is simply a wave in the ocean that is Spirit, no more or less important than the ocean itself—they are one.

Seeing itself as separate is an illusion that can either lead to the individual ego believing it is more powerful than it is, or believing it lacks strength because it is disconnected from any greater source of power. For example, the stereotypical "egomaniac" can be arrogant in a way that lacks the innocence I referred to previously, sometimes as a "self-made" person, perhaps with little respect or compassion for others. Her or his need for control is blatantly self-serving.

A second attitude that reflects an over-inflated ego is the person who feels so responsible for others, he or she becomes co-dependent or martyr-like. This person sees others as too weak, too sensitive, or too troubled to find their own way and so feels a need to take control of their lives, usually under an umbrella of denial called "I'm just trying to help you." This person can't see the bigger picture of other people's capacity to find their own path in life with more limited and appropriate support. Often, the person who consciously sees her/himself as serving others is actually feeling and acting superior.

At the other end of the continuum, an underdeveloped ego can damage our ability to shape, in the Human realm, the inspiration we receive from the Heaven realm. Again, different attitudes can prompt different responses in an underdeveloped ego. The ego can need a lot of approval, similar either to a child who always tries to be "good" or one who acts out to get attention. Either way the behavior doesn't arise from a grounded place.

Another result of a weak ego is that it can result in low self-esteem, preventing a person from valuing the gifts he or she has. For myself, there are certainly times when, even after so many years of practice, I have questioned my own authority or even my right to express my personal interpretation and application of Taoist concepts and to allow the *Way of Joy* to expand. Even though I developed this system myself, I have encountered my own glass ceiling. Stuck in the trappings of ego—the self-doubt, the fear that I'm a very poor vessel for conveying information that feels so vital to me—I can sabotage my own calling.

I believe it is particularly challenging for people who have been oppressed because of factors such as gender, race, sexual orientation, and age to maintain a healthy ego. For example, it can be excruciatingly difficult for women to experience the value of the "I-am-ness" I describe as ego, especially in a society that has traditionally expected women to know their place, to stay small. I have heard countless stories where talented and innovative women have hesitated to put their message, skill, or expertise forward, believing they just needed a little more education, a little more outside validation before taking that risk. And, if women or others who have been devalued by society do exert their creative power, they may often feel guilt and shame and see their own positive contribution in a negative light, as having too much ego.

Ego also plays a large role when we see the world as polarized opposites of "right or wrong." Once our ego starts to defend itself, we lose our grounding and engage in conflict, whether it is intellectual, emotional, spiritual, or physical.

Ego can get over-inflated during periods of expansion and deflate during times of contraction. Whether we're more inclined to have a puffed-up ego or a diminished one, the erratic swing of the pendulum can seem to be completely beyond our control and can damage us emotionally. The functioning of ego as a healthy connection to spirit becomes destabilized.

How do we not allow ego to be deceived into thinking it is an authority or the parent of the Self, responsible for (or capable of) running the show? At the same time, how can we, as individuals formed by all the elements of personality, enjoy ego and let ourselves accept the sense of identity it can give us?

While the answer to these questions isn't easy, I believe that a key to the solution lies in being able to move more gracefully in our cycles from expansion to contraction and back again. To do so can reduce shame for those who struggle with low self-esteem and give those prone to arrogance time to reflect and learn lessons that temper an inflated ego's sense of self-importance. The goal is to be conscious, even during cycles of expansion and contraction, that we are simultaneously the wave and the ocean. When we are able to do this, our ego can give us security, as our link to the ocean of universal power, and be a tool for creative expression.

Two Egos Talking

The body is a precious temple; honor your ego as the conduit of learning the soul.
—Ram Dass

I recorded a conversation I had with my partner, Sherry Mouser, in which she offered some comments on the nature of ego that I found valuable. Here is a partial transcription of that discussion.

Sherry: *I think there's a difference between calling and destiny, which is an expectation of a manifest pre-determined reality. Instead of destiny, I think ego is actually a calling. If I honor that calling, am mindful of it, stay in the process of fulfilling it, evolving it, then I'm in a state of joy. Although I may never ever do some of the things that I visualize, if I stay in the process of moving towards them, then I'm going to be fulfilled.*

It would make sense that each person comes in with their own blueprint in connection with Source and creates a personal vision of how that might manifest—some as teachers, some as healers, some as scientists, or whatever. It is like being a piece of the puzzle. Where's your right place? But it's not about how can I fit in with what is out there, but rather, how do I follow my own path and still stay in the present moment without being attached to a picture that has to look a certain way or have a specific kind of outcome.

Vicki: *That's where attachment to ego comes in, I think. Where we have* *a particular picture of where we are going and if it doesn't look that way, then we have failed. That's an ego construct.*

Sherry: *Well, it's an unhealthy ego construct. To me, the ego is like a tool, like a little utility in a computer that helps us live as physical beings because it holds the structure of information that gives us direction. Ego helps me move through the world of matter, while contributing to the non-tangible, universal pool of energy and consciousness that we all draw from.*

Maybe ego is God's way of staying entertained. If God is the total infinite everything, then maybe one way God gets to have fun is to create little aspects of self—it's a self-initiated jigsaw puzzle. Actually, I think of God as being not static but as constantly evolving, not only inspiring us as individual beings, but also being shaped in part by the contributions we each offer to the whole.

Vicki: *Ego is a gift that we've been given as a means of expression and I think we are meant to enjoy it. It's a gift to be in a body, to be alive.*

Conclusion: My Belt Test in Balance

When I first decided to take a sabbatical from teaching and left my *Way of Joy* Chi Kung school and beloved students to move to the country and write this book, my decision came from an inner drive I experienced as being beyond a calling—more like a spiritual imperative. The first few months were like a dream come true as the information I had been teaching for so many years began to coalesce into a structure that would become this book. My personal practice deepened as I became my only student, as I listened for guidance in meditation, walked the trails in the woods, and wrote.

It was literally when I began to think and write about the first Principle, *Balance Brings Harmony,* that the "interruptions" I described in the Prologue began to unfold—the serious illnesses and/or deaths of five people so close to me. It felt like the universe was giving me an unrelenting succession of belt tests that pushed me in physical, emotional, mental and spiritual ways to walk my talk.

I had to ask myself over and over during those first five or six months of cascading misfortunes, "What does balance mean, not just in the daily chaos of our lives, but also in facing profound instances of loss—those times in our lives that feel catastrophic? How can I be in harmony as I balance my attention to the people I love and to this project so close to my heart?" My initial impulse was to shout, "I have no idea! I feel like Job!"

I moved in and out of feeling victimized by events that were beyond my control. When I moved out of feeling helpless to a place of acceptance, I was able to tap into joy, that life force that sustains and informs us.

I heard myself saying, "Pay attention to your practice of balance on all four levels—physical, emotional, mental and spiritual, day to day, moment to moment." I asked myself and would hope for you, even in the most challenging days, to:

Physically—Breathe. Release tension with big sighs. Tend to your body. Watch what you eat, remember to stretch and do your Chi Kung. Notice when you are tired, or your body aches. Take time to rest and replenish, to walk in Nature, to get your blood moving. Monitor energy as it goes out, as it comes in, and remember to store some in "the bank." Remember that taking this time is most important when you have the least time for it.

Emotionally—Listen to your feelings, give time to grieve, rage, celebrate and laugh. As you process your emotions, allow them to flow freely from one to another and stay away from activities of the mind that want to analyze or rationalize. Pay attention to where you feel resolved with letting go and where you don't. Honor both.

Mentally—Observe your reasoning. Are you in the "victim mind-set," thinking that the world is doing something to you? Are you rationalizing that you don't have any healthy choices? Make sure your reasoning is about what you *can* do, rather than obsessing about what you *can't* do.

Behaviorally—Notice when you are drained and learn to say "no" with as much grace and celebration as "yes." Listen for when to let go and surrender and when to become pro-active. Pay attention to what you choose to do for others. Balance those choices with what you do for yourself. Offer what you can and stay humble. Learn whenever, whatever you can.

Spiritually—Balance time for meditation and prayer with times of service. Stay mindful and focus your attention on where you are, not on where you think you should be. Remember to trust that there will always be a time to expand, as well as a time to contract.

My experience deeply reinforced the principle of *Balance Brings Harmony*. I learned that it isn't possible for me to live in balance unless I embrace all of my life. Accepting everything in our lives without feeling like a victim requires that that we live in the balance of ego and higher Self, between the limits of our human understanding and our ability to tap into an awareness of greater Wisdom. When we do so, we can find the strength we need to remember that even when we are entranced by the often-intense narratives of any particular day, of any given moment, there is a larger picture. We don't need to "overcome" our human experience. Rather, we can enhance it.

In this state of balance, we will be able to ride our ocean of feelings like a surfer, remember the ocean for the waves, and so experience wholeness. In a society that clamors for us to "produce, produce, produce," we can give ourselves the time to experience a state of yin where we consciously receive both from others and from ourselves. Then, as we transition in a natural cycle, balancing back and forth between yin and yang, we can maximize our human potential for creativity and fulfillment. In this way we can live in accord with the Law of *Within Motion, Stillness; Within Stillness, Motion*, and find harmony in the balance.

CHAPTER 5
The Walk of Joy

```
        HEAVEN TRIAD
      Wisdom / Consciousness

      Within Motion, Stillness
      Within Stillness, Motion

   Balance              Embrace
Brings Harmony          Wholeness
```

Embrace Wholeness (Tao)
Practice of the Heaven Triad

Only by trusting life, being open and available to it, can you ever taste delight. And being delighted simply means joyfully experiencing the unexpected.
—Ma Deva Padma

The bride and groom, both graduate students at the university, held their wedding reception in their small apartment in the married student housing complex, an old transformed World War II army barracks. The mother of the groom, Adelina, came from Mexico for the wedding. Sharon, a friend of the bride, told me that although she and Adelina hadn't been able to converse because neither spoke the other's language, she'd been instantly impressed with Adelina's vibrant spirit. Shortly after the band began playing, Adelina walked past Sharon, who was standing near the door. Adelina passed her, observed her, their eyes met and held. Sharon felt such a deep sadness in Adelina that it radiated through her own body. Instinctively, trusting the bond she felt with Adelina, she followed her out onto the porch. Once there, tears welled up in Adelina's eyes and she began to sob. Silent, Sharon stayed with her, offering only the comfort of her presence as the woman began to wail. Adelina sobbed before she quieted, then turned to Sharon and embraced her in a long, heart-felt hug.

The band was playing a lively tune when Sharon followed her back in. With an exuberant "YaHAAAAA!" the woman slapped her knee and began to dance with a profoundly soul-filled spirit that merged a freedom and grace Sharon says she's never forgotten. Adelina danced the rest of the evening, irrepressible and joyful. Later, describing to the bride what had happened, Sharon learned that Adelina's only other son had died very recently.

I think Adelina is a beautiful model for how we might embrace the totality of life experience and enter the "dewy-eyed state" I referred to in the previous chapter. Once she gave herself the time and space to fully feel the grief of the unutterable loss of one son, she was able to experience the joy of her other son's wedding. By doing so, she became free, unencumbered in her merriment. Her "wholeness"—what I think of as her expression of the Tao—is in her ability to hold both extremes of sorrow and happiness in the same evening and in doing so fully embrace life in its complexity.

The coexistence and interdependence of opposites embedded in the Law *Within Motion, Stillness; Within Stillness, Motion,* and the application of that Law in the Principle, *Balance Brings Harmony,* leads us to the final aspect of the Heavenly triad—the Practice, *Embrace Wholeness* (or *Tao*). This Practice grounds the omnipresence of the Observer Self, an aspect that, despite always being present, we can easily forget or ignore. It lives and breathes within the inner stillness and balance available to us any time we choose to tap into it. To *Embrace Wholeness* means to cultivate ways to accept seeming opposites as interrelated, as Adelina did when she honored both her sadness and her joy.

An Introduction to the *Way of Joy* Practices

Life is something that happens while you're doing something else. The greatest tragedy in life lies not in how much we suffer but in how much we miss.
— Thomas Carlisle

As the Earth aspect of each triad, the general function of all of the *Way of Joy* Practices is to "bring it on home," where you take both the inspiration of the Law and the personalized interpretation of the Principle and ground them in your daily life. What follows in this chapter, as well as in the subsequent Practice chapters, is a variety of ways to integrate the meaning within the themes of each triad in practical and tangible ways in your daily life. In fact, the very names of the Practices themselves, *Embrace*

Wholeness, Cultivate Discernment, and *Allow Alchemy,* propose the kind of mind-set to take.

The Four Categories of Exercises Within the Practice

Each of the three Practice chapters has a series of exercises that guide and enhance your understanding of the three realms of Heaven, Human, and Earth. I have designed four categories of practical applications intended to direct your attention to how to live a joyful life: Embodying, Illuminating, Accessing, and Deepening.

1. *Embodying.* Embodying consists of the physical Chi Kung exercises through which I believe you will best viscerally experience the meaning contained within the Heaven, Human, and Earth realms. I've placed Embodying before Illuminating, Accessing, and Deepening because I strongly believe it is the foundation for all of the categories in the Practice. Whether or not you fully understand the Laws and Principles, the Chi Kung exercises create energetic patterns in your body that bring unexpected insights as well as an energetic flow, providing the foundation and springboard for a life based in joy.

If you practice the Chi Kung exercises when you read them, then by the time you reach the end of last Practice chapter, *Allow Alchemy,* you'll have a versatile range of Chi Kung tools to access and embody the energy of each of the three triads. In addition, at the end of *Allow Alchemy,* I've included a list of which Chi Kung forms I'd recommend for different challenging situations.

2. *Illuminating.* The next three categories support and enhance the information embedded in the foundational Chi Kung practices. "Illuminating" contains meditations and chants designed to enhance the visceral sense of each triad's themes that you initiated with your Chi Kung. These practices can be done sitting in a comfortable chair, on a meditation cushion (zafu), or lying down if you are unable sit for any length of time.

3. *Accessing.* This category contains life observation or awareness exercises designed to bring your attention to how joy can fuel you in "real time," that is, in literal and practical ways.

4. *Deepening.* Author Vita Sackville-West once said, "It is necessary to write if the days are not to slip emptily by." This category contains a series of short journaling exercises to explore each triad's themes more deeply.

While I recommend that you begin with the practices described in the "Embodying" category, feel free to do any of the exercises or categories in the order of your choosing. In fact, I don't want you to feel discouraged if you are not, at least initially, inclined to do all or any of them. I believe transformation can happen in many ways as you simply read this book.

Notice, as you look through the different exercises, which ones call up the most intense response. I recommend beginning either with the ones you are most drawn to or, if you are willing, the ones you feel most averse to. The main criterion is some kind of strong response. If you feel strongly drawn to a particular suggestion, go ahead and do that one. By the same token, if a suggestion seems unpleasant, try to not simply avoid it. Ironically, it is often the ones you feel most resistant to that will break open the biggest shifts in your awareness. On the other hand, if you simply feel open and curious about all of the exercises, then go through them one by one to explore whatever gift they might bring you.

Invoking the Wisdom of the Heaven Realm

All of the following exercises are designed to help you intentionally access your own wisdom and guidance, properties of the Heavenly triad. The purpose here is to remind you to shift from a dualistic, polarized perception of the world into one that is holistic, integrative, self-accepting and in an unwavering alignment with Source. In the days and weeks ahead, see if you can observe more closely how opposites, such as stillness and motion or expansion and contraction, appear in your life. As you do, you will cultivate and enhance your ability to hold the entirety of your experiences in a way that is essentially Taoist, all-encompassing and joyful.

Warm-ups/Stretches

Before you begin the Chi Kung practices, you might want to try a few of the following basic warm-up exercises. Although the subsequent Applied Chi Kung is quite gentle and may be done without these exercises, warm-ups are effective ways to relax and open your muscles and joints in order to maximize your experience of the flow of chi. Not drawn from traditional Chi Kung forms per se, these exercises are simply designed to get your breath flowing, your blood pumping, and your attention directed into your body. Some of them are taken from Taoist as well as other forms of Yoga, some from other martial arts, and others are stretches I have developed over the course of my years of teaching. You may do them for as little or as long as you like, staying with what feels good for your body at the time you are practicing. If you have an exercise/yoga/martial arts warm-up routine that you already enjoy, you are welcome to use it or to mix and match it with any of the suggestions below.

While you can start any stretch on either side, for the sake of clarity, the descriptions will always start on the right side, so I can delineate right and left movement.

Standing Stretches

Hip Circles: Drawn from almost every martial art, this exercise relaxes the lower back and gently opens up the hip joints. Stand with your feet hip distance apart. Place your hands on your hips and soften your knees so there is a very slight bend in them. Gently rotate your hips in a circle in one direction 9x. Then reverse and circle them in the other direction 9x. Allow your upper body to move in a slight opposition, so the hips are not isolated (as they might be in a belly dance kind of move), but rather so that your upper body counterbalances the movement of your hips.

Arm Circles: Circle your shoulders, moving them forward, then up towards your ears, back, then down 3x or more. Then place your hands on your shoulders and circle your elbows moving in the same pattern—forward, up, back, down—3x or more. Finally, drop both arms to your sides, and do a backstroke, circling one arm, then the other, forward, up, back and down.

Neck/Shoulder Release: Standing with your torso upright, let your head drop toward your right shoulder, stretching the left side of your neck. Do not force this position, but go as far as is comfortable. Then exhale as you gently extend the fingertips of your left hand down the side of your left leg, keeping your neck tilted to the right and your upper body vertical. Keeping your head tilted to the right, inhale as you relax the pull of the left hand. Repeat 3x or more. Next, let your head roll forward, chin towards the chest. Rotate your head from side to side as though you were saying "no" to a little bug on the ground. Gently and slowly straighten up through the back of your neck until you are completely vertical again. Then tilt your head to the left and repeat the exercise.

> **Variations:**
> 1. While your head is tilted to one side, circle the opposite shoulder slowly.
> 2. While your head is tilted to the side, rotate it to look down toward the ground, then up towards the sky.

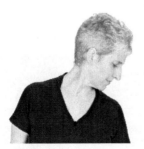
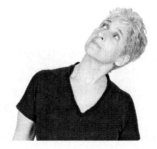

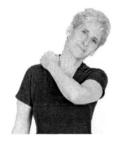

2. While your head is tilted to the right, make a fist with your right hand. Keeping your head tilted, cross your right arm over your chest to tap with that fist on top of your left shoulder, stimulating blood flow and warmth to that area.

Back of the Neck Release: Lace your fingers on the back of the base of your skull, over the occipital ridge (the "jade pillow"). Drop your chin to your chest, letting your elbows hang down with little to no pressure on the back of your neck. Then straighten your neck, raising your head back to vertical, drawing your elbows out to the side. Next, keeping your

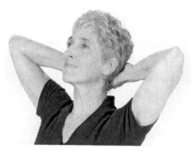

hands clasped on your neck, look up as you pull your elbows back, squeezing the shoulder blades together behind you. Repeat a few times.

Then lean forward, letting the top of your head hang down towards the ground. Starting at the back of the neck, lightly brush first one hand and then the other in a downward motion, from the base of your neck, down the back of your head (against the direction your hair grows), toward the ground, as if you were brushing something off the back of your head. Imagine you are removing any "brain mutter," anything that keeps you from being present, and let it drop to earth where it can compost.

Upper Back/Shoulders:

1. Bring your arms behind your back, hip level, and lace your fingers with your palms facing each other. Gently pull your hands down and back away from your body. While holding your arms in that position, turn your head to gaze back over your right shoulder. Repeat on the other side.

2. Lace your fingers in front of you at chest height, then rotate your palms so they face away from your body. Curl your upper spine back away from your hands, making your chest concave as though you were pushing back against a tree with your upper back. While in this position, move your arms to the right and take a moment to explore the stretch by moving your clasped hands around in space on that side. Do the same on the left.

3. Stretch your arms out to the sides at shoulder height, with your palms turned up. Squeeze your elbows towards one another behind your back and then stretch your arms out to the sides again.

Side and Back Stretches: Lift your right hand straight up towards the sky, letting your left arm dangle down by your side. As you inhale, imagine you are holding a bunch of balloons that are pulling you up, stretching your right side, until your heels can barely stay on the ground. Exhale and release the pressure, relaxing your arm. Repeat 3x or more. Then, leaning your torso to the left, stretch your right arm over your head to the left. Simultaneously, bend both your elbow and knees slightly, then straighten your knees and outstretched arm. Repeat 3x. Finally, with your arm still over your head, look to the left and down, rotating your head and upper torso to the left for a cross stretch across your back. Finish by hanging your upper body down in the center. Put your left hand on your left thigh, letting your right arm dangle in front of you. Circle your right arm a few times in each direction, as though you were stirring a big cauldron below you with your hand. Do the sequence again on the left side.

Back:

1. Bend your knees and lean forward, placing your hands on your lower thighs just above your kneecap and extending your back into an elongated "flat back." Curl your spine, rounding it up towards the ceiling as you drop your head, then arch your spine downward, lifting your head to look up in front of you.

2. Cross stretch. From the same flat back position, drop your right shoulder and twist your head to the left to look back over your left shoulder. Repeat on the other side.

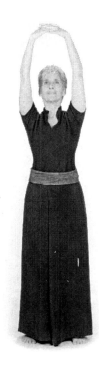

Hamstrings: These are called "Monkey Stretches." Lace your fingers and extend your arms toward the ceiling or sky with the palms turned down. Bending your elbows, move your hands slowly down the center-line of your body toward the ground, in front of your face, torso and legs as far as is comfortable for your legs and back. Then curl back up to vertical, bringing your arms back

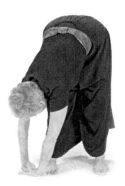 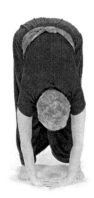

over your head. Turn your torso to the right, and repeat, bringing your palms down in front of your face and torso and continuing down toward the ground or your foot. Curl back up to vertical and turn to the left side and repeat. Perform this sequence of three stretches 3x or more, going from center, then to one side, then the other. **Note:** Don't push yourself to touch the ground; just go as far as your back and legs allow.

Calves/Feet: Place your right foot forward, and left foot back, keeping them about hip distance apart. Imagine you are standing on two parallel tracks, one under your right foot and the other under your left foot. This is a classic martial arts "forward stance." Bending your front knee, put about 70% of your weight forward. Straighten your back leg. Keep your torso vertical.

> **Variations:**
> 1. Keeping your weight 70% forward, lift and lower back heel.
> 2. Keep your back heel up and 70% of your weight in your forward foot. Bend and straighten your back knee.
> 3. Keeping your back knee bent, lower and lift your back heel. Bend and straighten your back knee while keeping your back heel on the floor.

Lying Down on your Back

Here are a few more warm-ups you can do lying on your back either in addition to the ones above or as alternatives to them.

Hamstrings: Begin with both knees bent, feet on the ground, near your buttocks. Raise your right leg straight up into air, keeping the other foot on the ground. Flex your top foot. Keeping your tailbone connected to the floor, grounded and stable, slightly bend and straighten your raised leg.

> **Variation:** Rotate right leg (from the hip) out to side, bend and straighten. Change legs.

Lower back: Bend your knees into your chest. Hug them in with your hands. Rock your weight forward and back, then side to side.

Hip: Begin with both knees bent, feet on the ground, near your buttocks. Cross your right ankle over your left thigh, just above the left knee. Rock from side to side, feeling a gentle stretch in the hip. If this feels easy, try bringing up your supporting leg (keeping it bent or extending it straight up), and rock side to side. You can hold on to the supporting leg with your hands or not, whichever feels more comfortable. Take your time, and if an area feels especially good to stretch, pause at that point in the rocking and move your supporting leg around gently to explore the stretch in the opposite hip. Repeat the process with your left leg.

Mid-back - Basic Cross Stretch: Lie flat on your back with your arms extended out on the floor, at shoulder height, palms up. Leave your right leg straight and bend your left knee, placing your foot on the ground near your right knee. Cross your bent knee over the right leg down toward or onto the ground. Turn your head to gaze back at your left arm. If your shoulder and knee do not touch the ground simultaneously, rock back and forth first letting your knee touch the ground, then the back of your shoulder.

Hands and Knees

Back: "Cat/Cow"

1. Position yourself on your hands and knees. Make sure your knees are directly under your hips and your hands are directly below your shoulders. Round your back up towards the sky, letting your head drop so that your whole spine is curved upwards. Then reverse the position, allowing your spine to arch down so it's relaxed in a sway back and hanging like a hammock while you simultaneously lift your head up.
2. Keeping your spine curled up like a hissing cat, gently shift your weight forward towards hands, then back towards knees.

The remainder of this chapter covers the four successive categories of exercises—Embodying, Illuminating, Accessing and Deepening.

Embodying the Wisdom of the Heaven Triad with Applied Chi Kung

Our bodies communicate to us clearly and specifically, if we are willing to listen to them.
— Shakti Gawain

One of the joys of Chi Kung is that as you intentionally move your chi, or life force, you are literally initiating change on a cellular level. While much has been written about the medical applications of these energy-based exercises, Chi Kung also has the capacity to create transformative shifts that reach beyond the physical plane. These shifts include but are not limited to

• A greater sense of inner peace
• The empowerment to initiate and sustain major changes
• The ability to stay calm, grounded, centered and focused, regardless of what is happening
• A renewed way of waking up in the morning ready to embrace what lies ahead, and
• A visceral sense of being more than a physical being, but rather, in fact, an embodied spirit.

In the end, all of these changes might be termed medical in that they could be considered vital aspects of good health. Traditional Chinese Medicine does not tend to distinguish these different levels of experience in the ways we do in the West.

The following tools can be used for a variety of applications. As you practice the following *Way of Joy* Chi Kung forms, you'll find yourself relying less and less on your will or the need to muscle your way through an intention in order to manifest what you want. In other words, rather than feeling as though you need to be a taskmaster in your life, you'll be enhancing the magnetism of your energy so that you attract more of what you want. This means even when you are not consciously trying to "make something happen," change will already be occurring on an energetic level through the movement of chi.

What follows are three forms to embody each aspect of the Heavenly Triad—the Law or inspiration, the Principle or interpretation, and the Practice or how you walk the talk. As you practice these forms, keep your attention half on what's happening inside of you, half on what's happening around you. Remember the principle you are working with here is *Balance Brings Harmony,* and by balancing your attention both on the inside and out, or yin and yang, you will find your way into the mind/heart set of the Law, *Within Stillness, Motion; Within Motion, Stillness.*

Stance: Modified Horse Stance

Many of the Chi Kung forms in this book are done in what is called a Modified Horse Stance. Sometimes the feet are parallel, sometimes very slightly turned out. The parallel stance is essentially yang, useful for forms where you are initiating change. The stance with feet slightly turned out opens the yin channels on the insides of the legs, so it is useful for when you want to receive a certain energy. I will offer recommendations for the stance for each form as you learn them; however, the main priority is to feel relaxed and at ease on your legs and feet. If you have a disability that restricts your movement or causes you pain, you can do any of the following forms sitting in a chair with or without arms. If you are in a wheelchair, adapt the movement in any way that feels comfortable or appropriate for you.

1. Stand with your feet parallel, about hip distance apart.
2. Lift your toes off the floor, spread them out and relax them back down to the ground so your feet feel wide, spread out like paws.
3. Relax the space behind your knees.
4. Stand as though the bones of your skeleton are stacked in perfect equilibrium, as though your ability to stand comes from this

delicate balance of one bone on top of another as much as by muscles holding you vertical. Standing becomes as effortless as possible.

5. Feel a connection between your sitz bones and your heels. Focus on your bubbling wells points[1] in your feet and visualize roots extending from these points three feet down into the earth.

6. Lift the crown of your head towards the sky, as though you were being pulled up like a sunflower opening to the sun. Imagine yourself responding to a magnetic draw from above at the same time you feel the pull of gravity from below. Feel yourself to be suspended between Heaven and Earth.

7. Relax your jaw. Allow there to be some space between your upper and lower teeth. Place the tip of your tongue on the roof of your mouth behind your front teeth. Relax the space between your eyebrows.

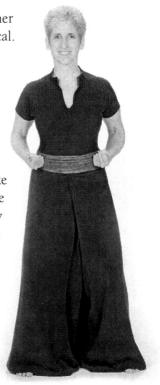

Chi Kung to Embody the Law
Within Motion, Stillness; Within Stillness Motion

Eye of the Storm

Eye of the Storm is a simple Chi Kung exercise that cultivates and increases your ability to embody the Law of *Within Motion, Stillness; Within Stillness, Motion*. With this form, you will practice being at peace, quietly centered in the face of chaos, regardless of what is happening around you— in other words, the stillness inside of motion. At the same time, you are practicing allowing the motion of your breath to live at the heart of that stillness.

In the martial arts, practitioners train to remain calm, centered, relaxed and engaged, regardless of what their opponent may be doing. On any given day, you may find yourself in a situation where you feel as though you have an opponent the size of a sumo wrestler throwing you off guard, disrupting your intention, impeding your direction, interrupting your flow. This experience may come from some external pressure that needs attention, such as your teenager demanding the use of your car even though you need to go grocery shopping or your boss wanting 25 things done *right now.* Or your opponent could be more internal, for instance when you're trying to decide what to do about a relationship you are dissatisfied with ("I don't know how to stand up to her—she's just impossible!") or how you are going to prioritize the activities of your day ("I have a million things going on—I don't even know where to begin!"), or something else that makes you anxious and restless. Whether the pressure you are feeling is internal or external, the impact is a sense of chaos or overwhelm. Your "opponents," be they demanding children and bosses or your own internal critics, keep you from being centered, from hearing your own guidance, from feeling the alive presence of Source, Wisdom, the Heaven realm in your life.

The purpose of *Eye of the Storm* is not to shut out or avoid the chaotic nature of life. Rather, you are practicing maintaining a state of inner stillness while staying connected to the world around you, thus enhancing your ability to respond in ways that best serve you instead of reacting in ways that do not.

The Form

1. Begin by turning your palms up and making fists with your hands. Bend your elbows, and bring them back until your upturned fists touch each side of your body, solar plexus height.

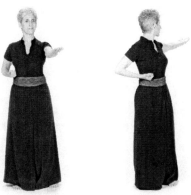

2. *Exhale —*

Physical: Keep the left elbow bent and left fist closed by your side. Open your right fist, the palm facing up, and, leading with the fingertips, stretch your right arm across your chest all the way past your left side. Reach through your fingertips as you exhale.

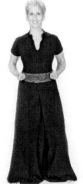
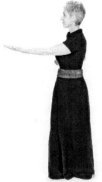

Focus: Focus your eyes on your fingertips.

3. *Inhale —*

Physical: Keeping your right arm at about chest (heart) level and parallel to the ground, palm up, sweep your outstretched arm back in front of you in a semi-circle. Then turn your waist to the right, stretching your hand behind you as far as you can go and still be comfortable.

Focus: Continue to watch your fingertips. Notice that as you move your arm, your fingers appear to be still as the world around you seems to move in the opposite direction. Notice the area just beyond the tips of your fingers where the apparent stillness of the hand and the moving space inter-connect.

4. a) *Exhale* —

Physical: Turn your waist back to center, bringing your right arm back until your hand is outstretched directly in front of you, pointing straight ahead, chest height, palm up.

Focus: Continue to gaze at the tips of the fingers and the apparent movement of the room.

   b) *Continue to exhale.*

Physical: Bend your right elbow so your fingers point up. Then drop your hand to elbow height, turning your palm down as you simultaneously reach forward. When your arm is extended in front of you, palm down, make a fist with your hand as though you were grasping the rim of a horizontal wheel you have just formed around you as you moved through the entire sequence.

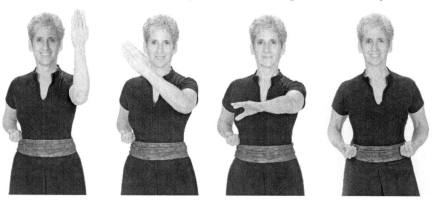

5. *Inhale* —

Physical: Turning your fist so the palm is up, draw your elbow back until your upturned fist touches the side of your body, solar plexus height. You have now returned to the position you started from.

Focus: As you make your fist, imagine that you are grasping the interconnection between your stillness and the whirling room. Breathe in the quality of stillness as you remain centered in the face of chaos.

6. *Exhale* —

Repeat the same sequence with the left hand going in the opposite direction.

Guidelines

As you practice, keep your attention half on what you are feeling inside your body, half on what you perceive around you. Keeping your eyelids slightly closed can help you suspend yourself between internal and external. Imagine that you can see/sense a horizontal circle surrounding you. Throughout the form, keep your eyes lightly focused on the spot where the fingertips and the spinning space seem to meet, where your inner stillness and the apparent chaos of the outside world interrelate. As you draw your arm back in, you will bring in the ability to stay present with the various kinds of stimuli the outside world brings to you at the same time you remain centered and grounded.

Again, this exercise is not about escaping from or shutting out the tumult. Rather, you are enhancing your ability to stay present with it without losing either your calm or your integrity.

Chi Kung to Embody the Principle *Balance Brings Harmony*

Lotus Balance

Lotus Balance balances the two sides yin and yang. It is particularly helpful when
- You are feeling physically or emotionally out of balance
- Your life feels out of balance, where your internal reality feels disparate from your external one
- You feel like you are juggling too many things in your life, or
- You feel like you want to place yourself in alignment between Heaven (guidance) and Earth (grounding).

The Form
Preparation: Stand in a *Modified Horse Stance* with your feet parallel. Place your palms on your lower *tan tien* with your left hand covering your

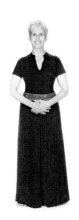

right. Close your eyes and breathe. Imagine you have a line going down the center of your body, separating your right side from your left. Take a moment to observe how the two sides of your body feel. Does one side feel tighter or more dense than the other? Does one side feel lighter? Is one shoulder higher, one hip lower? Do you have pain or discomfort on one side or the other? Notice whatever you notice, feel whatever you feel.

Physical

1. Move your hands out of the *tan tien* position, extending them in front of you with your elbows slightly bent. Turn your right palm up at hip level and your left palm down at collarbone level.

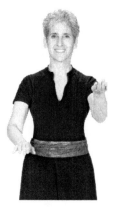

2. Simultaneously, move the lower hand up to collarbone height and the upper hand down to hip height so they have reversed levels.
3. Turn both hands over so the upper palm faces down and the lower faces up.
4. Again, move the lower hand up as you move the upper hand down, reversing levels.
5. Do this exercise at least 9x. Or continue for a longer time if you prefer or when you are feeling out of balance in any aspect of your life.

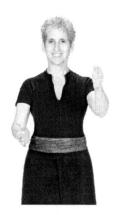
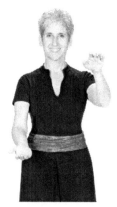

Breathing

If you choose, you may exhale as your hands change level and inhale as you turn your palms. However, if this does not feel natural or comfortable, breathe in any way you choose. The main instruction is to breathe in a relaxed and even manner.

General Focus

Feel for the weight of the air in your palms. Notice if the sensation is different between the two palms as you move them simultaneously. Does the density change when you lift one hand up from when you bring it down?

Imagine that your fingertips are stroking the texture of the air, as though it were a material like velvet, silk, or corduroy. Notice if you can feel the currents of air as they move around you.

Now bring your attention to your spine. Feel (or imagine you feel) energy traveling up one side of your spine and simultaneously traveling down the other side. Imagine that it is this movement on the two sides of your spine that brings your hands up and down, rather than your arm muscles—as energy travels up one side of your spine, your hand raises. As the energy descends on the opposite side of your spine, your hand lowers.

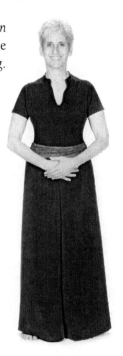

Close: Place your hands once again on your lower *tan tien* (lower abdomen), left hand over the right. Notice the two sides of your body. Notice your breathing. Check in to see if the two sides feel any different than when you checked before doing the exercise. If you feel an increased sense of balance between the two sides, take a moment to appreciate yourself for increasing your sense of well-being. If you do notice some differences, but still feel out of balance, try doing the exercise for another round of 9x, keeping your focus simply on your breath, relaxing your attention. Do *not* try to fix anything, but stay present with the movement itself. Then check in again. If you still do not notice any differences, try doing the form lying on your back, with your knees bent and feet placed near your buttocks. This can help align your spine, especially if you are compensating for pain.

Chi Kung to Embody the Practice *Embrace Wholeness*

The Shower

The *Shower*[2] integrates all three aspects of the Heaven triad and imbues the very cells of your body with inspiration and guidance—the large perspective. Here, you invite a larger worldview, the cosmic consciousness of Heaven, into your daily life. As you practice this form, you draw into your being the wisdom and integrity of the Observer on every level—physical, emotional, mental and spiritual—as you embrace the Tao and the qualities of the entire triad:

> Heaven (stillness in motion)
> Human (balance and harmony)
> Earth (manifestation and wholeness)

The Form

Stand in *Modified Horse Stance* with your feet slightly turned out to open the *yin* channels on the insides of your legs. You will be circling your arms up and around your body.

1. Open your arms out to the side, palms facing up.

2. Lift your arms, palms up, until you imagine holding a little cloud about 6 inches above your head.

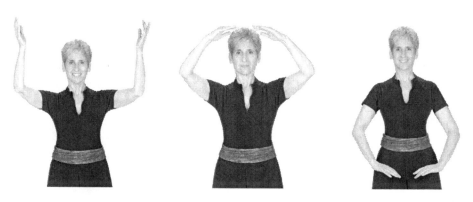

3. Continue the circle by pressing your hands down in front of you, palms down, to just below your hips.

4. Practice 3-9x.

Steep the Tea

After you have completed your Chi Kung practices, take a moment to "steep the tea"[3] by lying down on your back and allow the energy you have engendered to simply move through you. See if you can do nothing but rest, allowing the "tea" of your efforts to "steep" into your consciousness. If your mind begins to go into overdrive (as it so often does when we stop "doing"), put your attention on your breath as it moves in and out, and relax your mind. You might try thinking the words, "I am breathing in" as you inhale and "I am breathing out" as you exhale. Alternately, you can try counting to 4 as you inhale and 4 as you exhale. What you do with your mind is less important, however, than simply allowing your body to rest and take in on a cellular level whatever information and benefits you have received from your Chi Kung practice. After you have rested on your back for a few moments, turn onto your side and curl up into a little ball. Breathe into your spine for a few more moments before getting up.

Tapping It In

This exercise takes one final step after *Steeping the Tea* to assimilate the chi you have moved with your Chi Kung. Many of the different Chi Kung systems I have encountered over the years have some form of tapping exercise to stimulate and awaken the meridians. I suggest you do the exercise as a way to tap into your body any useful information from your Chi Kung practice.

1. Stand comfortably with your feet hip width apart. Beginning with your left hand, pat your hand lightly on your chest, over your breastbone (and thymus gland).

2. Pat over the front of your right shoulder and over the top of it. Continuing to pat down the outside of your right arm, tapping the back of your right hand, then your palm. Then continue to pat up the inside of your arm up to the armpit and then back to the center of your chest.

3. Change hands so the right hand takes over patting the center of your chest and do the same process on the other side, using your right hand to pat down the outside of your left arm and up the inside of it to your armpit and back to your chest.

4. Continue the rhythm of your patting as you bring both hands to pat the chest, then pat down the front of the body, over the solar plexus and belly. Then separate the hands and pat your way to the outside of your hips.

5. Pat the outside of your hips and buttocks. Lean forward, bending your

knees, if you like, to keep your back comfortable and continue to pat down the outsides of your legs, from your thighs all the way down to your ankles and over the tops of your feet.

6. Pat the insides of your legs, moving up from your inner ankles all the way up your inner thighs.

7. Move your patting now to your lower back and pat up your back over your kidneys, moving up as high as is comfortable for your shoulders.

8. When you have patted as high as you can on your back, bring your arms back in front of you and pat the tops of your shoulders.

9. With your fingertips, now tap up and down the back of your neck and then behind your ears.

10. Finish by tapping lightly all around the top of the crown of your head.

11. When you have finished, clap your hands in the air over the top of your head and then rub them together briskly, generating some warmth in your palms. Move your palms down your face and continue down the front of your body. You can either keep legs straight or bend your knees as you slide your hands down in front of your legs all the way to your feet. *Go only as far as is comfortable for your back.*

12. Next, circle your hands to the backs of your heels and move them from the heels up the backs of your legs then as high as you can up your back. When you've gone as far up as you can on your back, simply move your arms to the front of your body, then reach your fingertips behind your neck so they slide up the back of your neck and head. Brush briskly up, as though you were flicking something off the back of your head. Repeat 2x more.

13. With your hands at face level, imagine you are splashing water onto your face. Use a scooping motion to get the water as you would from a basin of water in front of you, then brush your hands in a splashing motion towards your face until you feel the air move against your skin, "waking yourself up." (see footnote 3)

Illuminating the Wisdom of the Heaven Triad

What follows are two guided meditations based in the Heaven triad. You will find there are several different ways you can enter the meditations throughout this book. Here are a few suggestions. Feel free to adapt any of them in whatever ways best suit you.

You will need a comfortable chair or cushion to sit on. If you cannot sit comfortably, you may lie down. You may choose to have a journal or notebook and pen.

1. On your own: First read the entire meditation through to yourself, either silently or out loud. Then re-read part 1. Close your eyes and picture the image. Once you are able to feel, sense, or see it, open your eyes, keeping your internal focus, and read the next part. Stay aware of your breath as you read, then close your eyes and enter part 2.

2. Ask a friend to read the text to you as you meditate: Ask the friend to read each part slowly and clearly as you sit with eyes closed. Be sure to let the person know when you are ready to move on (by saying "OK" or using a hand signal) or if you would like any part read more slowly (by raising your hand).

3. Taped: If you'd like to do the meditations without having to read as you go, you can record yourself reading the meditation. Leave a pause in-between each part so you can remain deeply relaxed as you move from one part of the guided visualization to the next.

To begin all meditations:

When you sit for your meditation, it's important that your spine be comfortable and aligned. If you're accustomed to meditating, you may choose to sit in your usual position. If you don't already have a regular sitting practice, you may either sit on the floor on a cushion or zafu, or you may choose to sit in a chair. Be sure your position does not impose any undue physical strain or make you uncomfortable. If you are using a chair and need extra support for your back, place a pillow behind you so that your spine is supported. Regardless of your physical condition, take the time to discover how to keep your spine vertical so that your sitz bones feel grounded.

As I mentioned, if you're uncomfortable sitting, you may choose to do these meditations lying on your back, placing a cushion under your knees to keep your lower back relaxed. The only danger here is that you may fall asleep. If you do, allow yourself to drift, rest well and try the guided meditation another time sitting up, or when you are not as likely to fall asleep. If you do fall asleep, please know this is not a problem. In fact, studies show it's sometimes in sleep that we best assimilate what we've learned.

Whether you're seated on a chair or lying on your back, keep your knees in alignment with your hips and send chi down your shins to your feet. If you're seated cross-legged on a cushion, imagine the energy traveling through your legs down to your bubbling wells (kidney 1) points. Imagine that you're grounding your energy through the bubbling wells into the earth. Picture your spine unfurling from your tailbone up through the second chakra in your belly, the third chakra in your solar plexus, the fourth chakra in your heart center, the fifth chakra in your throat, the sixth chakra at the third eye in the middle of your forehead, and finally the seventh chakra in your crown.

Be sure to relax the space between your eyebrows and your jaw. Lightly place the tip of your tongue on the roof of your mouth.

Candle Meditation

Intention

This first meditation is intended to stop your "brain mutter," the constant inner monologue so many people carry around inside their minds every moment of every day. The purpose here is to take time out from your problem-solving self and move into the present moment, thereby enhancing your ability to stay grounded and centered as you did with the *Eye of the Storm* Chi Kung form. Here you can access the Heavenly Law of *Within Motion, Stillness; Within Stillness, Motion* that leads you to your own guidance and inspiration.

Meditation

Part 1. Close your eyes and bring your attention to your breath. Take a moment to focus on nothing but the sensation of your breath as you inhale and exhale. Imagine that with each breath you enter into a place of deeper stillness. You have nothing to do but stay present with your breath. If your mind begins to wander to the events of the day or any other preoccupations, notice that is so, make an agreement with yourself to come back to those issues later and gently bring your attention back to your breath. Listen to the sound of the air moving as you inhale and exhale. Then, keeping your eyes closed, open your ears further and listen to the world around you. Hear whatever you hear and take in whatever information you take in. Keep your attention half on your breath, half on what you are hearing. Allow sound to pass through you without "listening," that is, without thinking about the sounds you hear, trying to identify them or give them some kind of story. If your mind wanders or begins "muttering," once again bring your attention back to your breath.

Part 2. Imagine there is a candle flame somewhere in your body. You might see it in your third eye, your heart, your solar plexus or your belly. Notice where it is. Feel the light, the heat. Breathe.

Part 3. As you inhale, imagine you are feeding oxygen to that inner flame. As you exhale, watch the flame and notice its flicker. Slow yourself down. Keep your breath even. Observe the candle flame becoming more robust as you breathe, warming you throughout your body.

Part 4. Ask yourself, if I could have this flame illuminate some aspect of my life, what would it be? Don't go into problem-solving or "how tos." Just stay with the image of the light of the candle gently shifting shadow into light, moving from what is obscure to what can be known.

Journal

Jot down any insights, images, impressions or thoughts you experienced.

Age and Youth or the Eternal Present

Intention

The purpose of the following visualization is to transcend the constraints of linear time and in so doing access wisdom and guidance from your future and past selves.

Meditation

Part 1. Entering the meditative space: If you'd like to review the body position, breathing, and mind clearing in preparation for this meditation, see instructions on page 97 to review.

Part 2. Imagine you are gazing at your reflection in a mirror. As you look into your eyes, picture yourself aging slowly, getting older and older, until the reflection you see is a future wiser self, perhaps a crone or an old wise man. Take some time to see this much older self gazing back at you. See where the laugh lines are, how your face might look many years ahead. As you gaze into those eyes, imagine you are entering deeper and deeper into them as a pebble dropping into a lake.

Part 3. Now imagine that you are shifting your consciousness from your present self into that future self who is looking back at you. What do you see as you look from the future at who you are today? What information do you have about the current events of your life? What would you like this "past" self to know? Listen deeply to any answers to these questions. When you feel done, continue to look at your present self from the eyes of the future.

Part 4. As you hold your gaze, now picture yourself becoming younger and younger until you see yourself as a child playing, doing something that you absolutely loved to do—an activity that was comforting, entrancing or just plain fun. Notice your energy, openness, spirit. Observe the qualities of your young vulnerable self that you love, admire, can appreciate. Notice what you feel as you watch this child and ask if she or he has any information for you, anything he or she wants you to remember in your present life. Listen to her answers.

Note: If you find yourself suddenly remembering trauma, ways in which you may have been hurt when you were young, take a moment to acknowledge that pain or sadness. Then ask yourself to agree, if you need to work with this issue, to do so at another time, perhaps in a journal, with a therapist or a trusted friend. Then, see if you can guide yourself to see a time when your child self was feeling comforted.

Part 5. Move back into the present self. Picture your old self holding the hand of your young self. Imagine that through their eyes, they are sending you the qualities, strengths, and energy they wish for you today. Receive it. Breathe.

Journal

Jot down any insights, images, impressions or thoughts or reactions you have experienced.

Three Realm Toning

With this meditation, through the vibration of sound, you will awaken and enliven energy in each of the *tan tiens* (energy centers) in your body: *Shen* (Heaven realm), *T'ai* (Human realm) and *Jing* (Earth realm). Vibrating the triple *tan tien* in this way keeps your cellular body well centered in the Human position aligned between Heaven and Earth.

This meditation may also be done sitting in a chair, on a cushion or the ground, or lying down, if needed.

Preparation and Guidance

For each of the chants, relax your throat and imagine the breath is coming from your belly to support the sound. If your throat starts to feel tight or to hurt, reduce the volume and sound the tone more quietly. You don't need to make the tone last for any particular amount of time.

Whatever amount of breath you have is the perfect amount. The same is true for the pitch (the note). You will chant on three different pitches: low, mid-range and high. There is no "wrong" note or sound. Use whatever pitch and volume is comfortable. Your intention is to use your voice to vibrate your bones.

Unless you are a singer or someone who already chants frequently, I would suggest you begin this practice by toning 3x into each of the three energy centers. Over time, as you become more comfortable and stronger using your voice in this way, you can increase the number of repetitions. The optimal number is 9x. The main point here is to avoid any strain. Take the time and energy that is comfortable and do the number of repetitions that feel right in order to enjoy the impact of the sound vibrations as you align your energy centers between Heaven and Earth.

The Chant

1. Start with the lower *tan tien*, the Earth realm in your body, also known as the center of your *Jing*. The energy center for your physical being, energy, stamina, this is the very matter of which your body is made.
   a. Focus on your sitz bones, your pelvis, legs and feet—your base. Imagine that you have roots extending from your tailbone down into the earth. What do you notice about your physical state of being at this very moment? Are you thirsty? Tired? Relaxed? Is your mind buzzing or quiet?
   b. Using the lower, deeper range of your voice, tone the syllable *om*. Feel the vibration of the sound traveling into the bones of your pelvis, legs and feet. Allow the sound to vibrate your whole body from the base up until you feel as though you are shaking any stagnation loose. After you have completed the sound, take a moment to pause and feel whatever you feel. Tone the sound 3–9x.
   c. After you have completed your repetitions, take a moment to notice how you feel in your body. Observe any sensations or impressions. Then ask yourself the following question: "Where in my life do I experience abundance and health? What gives me grounding and nourishment?" Take a moment to appreciate these sources. Breathe them into the cells of your body and your lower *tan tien*.
2. Move your attention to your middle *tan tien*, the Human realm of your body. The *T'ai* is your expression, your heart's desire, your unique voice. This is the energy center that holds the interconnectedness between you and the web of life.

   a. Take a moment to focus on your heart center, your chest and
      breastbone (sternum) in the front of your body and the area
      between your shoulder blades (scapulae) in the back. Imagine that
      your spine lengthens as the chest softens and relaxes. What do
      you notice about your emotional/ feeling state at the moment? Are
      you feeling connected to others? Are you hurt or angry? Do you
      feel tight in your chest, or does your breath move easily?
   b. Using the middle range of your voice, tone the syllable *haaah* into
      your chest and upper back. Allow the sound to vibrate the heart
      center of your body, listening for a buzz or tingling sensation in
      that area. Repeat 3-9x.
   c. Take a moment to notice what you feel in your chest. Observe any
      sensations, feelings, or emotions. Then ask yourself: "Where in
      my life do I experience joy? What people, places, thoughts, events
      and things do I feel an emotional connection with? What do I want
      to offer my family, my friends, my community, the planet?" Take
      a moment to experience those connections with whatever images
      occur naturally. Breathe them into the cells of your body.
3. Move your attention to your upper *tan tien*, the Heaven realm in your
   body. The *Shen* is your spirit, your guidance, the larger perspective, your
   connection to Source.
   a. Take a moment to focus on your neck, head and the top of your
      head at the crown. Notice if the bones of your head feel constricted
      or open. Do you sense a sense of spaciousness, or does your head
      feel dense or heavy? Notice if you feel a difference between the
      front of your head (behind the forehead) and the back.
   b. Using the high range of your voice, or *falsetto*, tone the syllable
      "sseeeeee" directing the sound into your head and lightly vibrating
      the bones of your skull 3-9x. (If you tend to get migraines, you
      may want to tone this sound very softly). Relax your jaw, allowing
      space between the upper and lower jaws. Place your attention on
      the space between your eyebrows and the crown of your head.
   c. When you are finished, take a moment to notice what you feel in
      your head. Observe any sensations, thoughts or images. Then ask
      yourself: "What are the ways in which I experience guidance in my
      life? What helps me hold a larger perspective? When is the last
      time I remember feeling aligned with my own greater purpose?
      Are there any images or thoughts that came to me during this
      chant that contain information that might be useful?"

At the end of this chant, take a moment to rest, place your attention on your breath and notice any tingling sensation you feel in the areas of *Shen, Taiji,* or *Jing.*

Accessing Wisdom of the Heaven Triad in your Daily Life

Sometimes your joy is the source of your smile, but sometimes your smile can be the source of your joy.
— *Thich Nhat Hanh*

Choose one of these exercises to practice throughout this next week. Then, over the next several weeks, try another observation exercise, then another. See if you can give each of exercises at least one week to play with. Take time at the end of each day to jot down some notes about your observations into your notebook or journal.

Accessing Stillness

Take a moment every now and then to stop whatever you are doing, whether at work or at home, and just breathe. Listen. What do you hear in the world around you? In yourself? See if you can maintain a moment of not-doing, staying receptive to whatever may be coming into your awareness as you practice being still in the midst of motion. Breathe into the center of that stillness.

Accessing the Witness

Several times a day, go into the place of stillness you practiced in the previous exercise. Now check in with your Observer Self. Witness what you are experiencing in your mind, heart, and body. Are you stressed or at ease? Is your body tight or relaxed? Is your mind racing? What is your brain mutter saying? See if you can simply notice whatever you notice without analyzing or going into problem solving, as though you were observing yourself in a dream. Notice what you are doing and how you are being. Detach and enjoy!

Accessing Wisdom

Once a day, take a moment to intentionally slow down your breathing. Take three long, deep inhalations, exhaling slowly. Ask yourself the question—"If guidance, an angel, or Higher Power were to speak to me at this very moment, what would he/she say?" Make a note of what you hear and put it on your bathroom mirror or someplace you will see it every day. As the messages accumulate, make a point of reading them daily.

Accessing Grounding

Take a moment to step outside or look out of your window and watch leaves move in the breeze, or look at a flower, bird, or other element of Nature. Breathe several deep breaths as you regard whatever you are seeing/perceiving. As you inhale, imagine Heaven energy coming into the crown of your head, then down through the centerline of your body into your feet. As you exhale, allow that energy to travel down three feet into the earth.

Deepening the Wisdom of the Heaven Triad: Journal Exercises

Following are several "rapid write" exercises, for which you will need your journal and a pen. The guideline for a rapid write is that you write for a prescribed amount of time, so you will also need a watch or timer, preferably with an alarm or beeper that you can set for a certain number of minutes.

I will suggest a starting phrase (which you are welcome to reword in any way that seems more appropriate to your circumstance). Write continuously without taking your hand off the page—whatever comes to your mind without censorship. You are not trying to create prose here, but, rather, training yourself to listen to your own guidance through your thoughts, impressions, and feelings. Even if at first all you hear are thoughts like "I don't feel like doing this exercise, I don't get it..." keep writing. You may want to write the opening phrase I have suggested over and over, making a list of responses. Or you may find yourself wandering into unrelated territory. Just keep writing, even it's about something that appears to be off-topic.

While writing on one prompt for 2-3 minutes may initially sound like a long time, in practice my students have often experienced that it often seems not quite long enough. In fact, continuing to free-write after you think you're "done" or get blocked can often take you to even deeper insights that may surprise you.

Write until the time is up and then stop. If you find you have only just begun, that you have more to say, you can always return to the exercise whenever you wish. However, the main idea for the initial exercise is to keep it brief.

The goal here is to strike a balance that allows you to go into a deeper place of inner listening, yet not be so extensive or complex that you end up sabotaging yourself and not doing the exercise because you do not have time or feel overwhelmed. See if you can make these times of journaling as effortless and pleasurable as possible.

You might try an exercise right before you go to bed or immediately after you wake up. If you keep your journal next to your bed, then you can just reach over for it. Or you might try writing after lunch before you get back to work. Find a time when you can give yourself approximately 3-10 minutes of your full attention. The intention here is to hear your own guidance, to be fully in your own good company.

To prepare, get into a comfortable position for writing, take a deep breath and set your timer. Then write the following phrases and fill in the blank. Try to write as you think, rather than stop and think, then write. Let your pen lead you.

Embrace Wholeness
Recommended Time: 3 minutes
For me to joyfully and wholeheartedly embrace my life and all that it brings, I would need to . . .

Call to Wisdom
Recommended Time: 3 minutes
I know I am connected to my guidance when I . . .

The Witness Speaks
Before you begin, take a moment to close your eyes and sit with your body aligned. Lift your crown towards the Heaven realm and ground yourself through your sitz bones. Imagine you are one with your Observer. Breathe and listen.

Recommended Time: 3 minutes
As the Observer, I want (put your name here) to know that . . .

Getting There
Recommended Time: 3 minutes
One of my favorite ways to access Wisdom is to . . .

Seeing the Pattern
This is a three-part rapid write to help you identify how you tend to behave after a large output of energy. The goal of the exercise is for you to become more aware of your own personal patterns of post-expansion contraction.

Recommended Time: 3 minutes for each part
>   1. *At the end of a big project I usually find I . . .*
>   2. *One thing this response robs me of is . . .*
>   3. *One thing this response gives me is . . .*

At the Completion of an Effort

Do this rapid write after you have actually completed something that took a good deal of effort, such as at the end of a long project. Write down each phrase and leave space to fill in the blanks.

Recommended Time: 3 minutes for each part
>   1. *Today I completed . . .I feel . . .*
>   2. *One way I can take in and acknowledge what I have accomplished is to . . .Another way is to . . .*
>   3. *What I most need now to replenish myself is . . .*

Balance Charts

The following two charts are designed to support you in observing how you are using your energy throughout the week.

Balancing Yin and Yang

Intention

This exercise examines how you currently balance your yang and yin activities. How do you extend your energy? How do you replenish yourself? Think of this exercise as an exploratory tool, rather than a "test" on how well you are doing, connecting with your Observer as you go through the week.

Exercise

Draw a line down the center of a page in your journal. On one side, write the word "OUT." On the other side, write "IN." Under the "OUT" column, make a list of everything you do that expends energy, such as chores like laundry or cooking a big meal. Or include a work project, dealing with a difficult co-worker or colleague, taking care of a sick family member, etc. Then, in the "IN" column, make a list of what feeds you, brings energy back in, such as quality time with a beloved or close friend, writing in your journal, eating a healthy meal.

After you've completed your "OUT" and "IN" lists, choose the top five in each category and enter them into the chart below. If you have more than five items you want to track, see if you can group them (see sample chart). You may find that at different times certain activities can be either yin *or* yang. For example, sometimes spending time with a friend is nourishing while at other times it's draining. In this case, you could enter the same thing under both categories "IN" and "OUT." Enter the days of the week into the top of the chart. Then each day, place a check mark or note in the box for that activity or choice. At the end of the week, notice how the two match up.

As you do this exercise, try to avoid judging yourself. This is not a "test" to see how "good" you are at taking care of yourself. Rather, it's a tool to evaluate what keeps you in your flow. How do you attend already to your well-being at the same time you take care of the demands in your life? You may find you are doing better on any given day than you'd have thought—or you may discover specific adjustments you could easily make that would enhance your balance.

The first chart is a sample of what you might do. The blank spaces indicate "didn't get to it," while a checkmark signifies that the task was accomplished. Some boxes have little notes detailing what was done in that particular category if you want to remember it rather than simply checking it off.

Following the sample chart is a blank chart for you to copy and use as a worksheet. Full-size blank worksheets are also available for printing at WayofJoy.com.

Example of Worksheet for Yin-Yang Balance

IN	Mon	Tues	Wed	Thurs	Fri	Sat	Sun
Chi Kung Meditation Chant	Whole Heavenly Triad 3x each form	Candle Meditation Shower 9x	Eye of the Storm 3x		Candle Meditation	Sat still for a few minutes this morning	
Fitness Aerobics Stretch	Brisk Walk in the park		gym		Yoga Class	Stretched a little	
Nature	Walked in park, saw red-tailed hawk				Sat outside and watched squirrels		Worked in garden
Entertainment Reading Movie		crossword puzzle	Read novel before bed			Dinner and movie with Elsa	Rented DVD and watched with kids
Being/Self Care Inner Listening Journal	Hot epsom salts bath	Thought: Expect inspiration in unexpected places	Ugh!	↘	Took notes on meditation	Doodled a picture	
OUT	Mon	Tues	Wed	Thurs	Fri	Sat	Sun
Work	↘	↘	Finished project with Alan	↘			
Chores Errands	Groceries Meal Prep	Kids to band practice Meal prep	meal prep	Timmy cooked! (with some help)		repaired lamp	cleaned gutters
Listen & Give attention to other(s)	Story time	↘	Story time Talked to Frank		Story time	Helped J figure it out	KIDS ALL DAY
Fitness Aerobics Stretch	Walk		gym			Stretched a little	
Creative Time					started a poem about squirrels		
NOTES for the day	Walk was replenishing; glad I did it				want to work on the poem daily		Fun day but tiring

Worksheet for Yin-Yang Balance

IN	Mon	Tues	Wed	Thurs	Fri	Sat	Sun			
OUT	Mon	Tues	Wed	Thurs	Fri	Sat	Sun			
NOTES for the day										

Way of Joy Chi Kung™

Embracing Yin

Intention

Given that so many people have the tendency to get trapped in a state of unending expansion with no internal space for contraction, I've constructed this chart to facilitate your awareness of how you experience yin.

As we saw with the "Balance of Three," in Chapter 4, both Khaleghl Quinn and Masaro Emoto suggest that in order to come to a place of balance, we need to be two parts yin to one part yang. If contraction is truly a time for self-nourishing, how can you build it into your schedule? What would that mean or look like? This exercise is particularly useful when you are feeling drained, depressed or aware that you aren't taking care of yourself well. Tracking your patterns in this way may not only help you evaluate the ways in which you already do or don't take care of yourself, but also will remind you on a daily basis of things you might do as well.

Exercise

Going back to the "IN" list you just made, choose 10 to 15 items that consistently replenish your energy and enter them into the chart below. You may want to add more ideas to the list you've already made. This does not mean that now you have to find (or make) even more time to try to fit "stuff" in every single day or week. Rather, look for choices that, *if* you made them frequently (or even occasionally), would sustain and replenish you—provide you with a sense of balance. You might add things like being sure to get to bed by 9 or 10 for a good night's sleep at least once a week. Or reading a book purely for pleasure. Or grabbing a few minutes to chant, meditate or practice Chi Kung. Or you might pull a divinatory card or open a sacred scripture for inspiration and guidance. Or go to the gym, spend time in Nature, or buy a new pair of shoes. You might go people-watch or pull out your camera and take pictures, renewing a love of photography. Or have dinner with a friend. (Studies show that people who see their friends actually live longer than those who don't. Yet how many of us can *think about* seeing a friend for months without doing it?)

However you choose, pick a variety of things that are for *you*, that are fun, inspiring, nurturing and/or relaxing, where you feel replenished. Remember, this exercise is to help you observe what you *are* doing, not to guilt trip yourself for things you think you *should* do, don't have time for, etc.

Again, I have made a sample chart. In this one, I used one example of doing Chi Kung daily, not to pressure you but to inspire you regarding what kind of impact a few minutes of Chi Kung might have if done regularly. (These exercises could take as little as 21 minutes per week or 3 minutes a day!) What other nurturing things in your life actually take such little time?

Follow the same system as the previous exercise. Every day, place a check in the boxes for choices you've made to take care of yourself. If you like, make notes to remind yourself of times you want to remember. Remember, you do not have to do everything on the list every day. Let the list be flexible—you may find you want to add or subtract things as you go along.

Following the sample chart is a blank chart for you to copy and use as a worksheet. Full-size blank worksheets are also available for printing at WayofJoy.com.

Example of Yin Observation Worksheet

IN	Mon	Tues	Wed	Thurs	Fri	Sat	Sun
Chi Kung	Eye of Storm	Eye of Storm	Eye of Storm	Eye of Storm	Lotus Balance	Embrace Wholeness	All 3 Heaven Triad Forms
Meditation Chanting Prayer	✓	3 realms	✓	✓	Age/Youth	Candle	
Self Nurture	Massage with Clara		Hot epsom salts bath with lavendar		Herbal tea before bed		
Journal	✓	✓	✓	✓	✓	✓	✓ Extra
Fitness Aerobics Stretch		Yoga class		took time to stretch	walked at Marina during lunch break		walked 2 miles in park
Time in Nature						garden	park
Reading	Artist's Way		great mystery	✓		✓	
Entertainment			A and I watched DVD "What the Bleep"			concert	
Food	No sugar today	oops, busy too much junk		began fat flush diet			good breakfast good energy
Sleep	in bed early	restless had trouble going to sleep	in bed by 10	woke up and wrote in middle of night	woke early ready to go in bed by 11	Slept in 10 hours Tea helped	in bed by 10
NOTES for the day	Big rain this evening, enjoyed reading in bed		Felt off this am but better this evening	Figured out what to do about Stan	Had good energy today got a lot done		Felt really rested today

Worksheet for Yin Observation

IN	Mon	Tues	Wed	Thurs	Fri	Sat	Sun
NOTES for the day							

Way of Joy Chi Kung™

Conclusion: Grounding the Heaven Triad

Take the first step in faith. You don't have to see the whole staircase.
Just take the first step.
— Martin Luther King, Jr.

When you choose to *Embrace Wholeness* (Tao), you move into a state of wisdom, an all-inclusive state of embodied Awareness, "trusting life, being open and available to it…joyfully experiencing the unexpected," as Ma Deva Padma says. This means being fully present with all-that-is without falling into the trap of polarities—good/bad, doing/being, expanding/contracting, etc.

The Observer Self is the center focus of the work done in all three aspects of this triad—the Law, the Principle, and the Practice. The Law of the Heaven triad, *Within Motion, Stillness; Within Stillness, Motion* teaches us that we are all manifestations of divine breath, so that when we inspire (draw in breath), we connect to our larger vision, creating a personal connection to the cosmos. It is through your breath that you find the stillness you need to access the Observer.

The insights you gain from your Observer Self become the context for how you express the Human aspect of the Heaven triad. The interplay of opposites, as polarities, becomes a dance of balance and interconnection prescribed by the Principle of *Balance Brings Harmony*.

In the Earth aspect of this triad, you live out both the Law that brings you to your Observer Self and the Principle that moves you beyond the divisions of polarization to the ability to access joy as your fuel. In this way, the Practice of *Embrace Wholeness* is the embodiment of conscious living, the Heaven triad incarnate.

PART II
The Heart of Joy
Intention

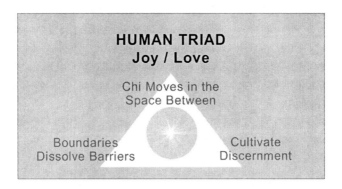

HUMAN TRIAD
Joy / Love

Chi Moves in the
Space Between

Boundaries   Cultivate
Dissolve Barriers   Discernment

I found God in myself and I loved her fiercely.
—*Ntozake Shange*

The Human triad of the *Way of Joy* contains the Law, Principle, and Practice that reflect each individual's expression of the other two triads. Residing at the center of the *Way of Joy* and emanating Love and Joy, the Human triad is where Heaven and Earth come together, where, as Ken Wilber says in his moving memoir, *Grace and Grit,* "Earth grounds Heaven and Heaven exalts Earth."[1] When Heaven and Earth are aligned through the Human realm, we experience a sense of peace, being in right time and place. Acting as a conduit between Heaven and Earth, between the macrocosm and the microcosm, between the infinite perspective of the cosmos and day-to-day reality, the Human triad holds our life purpose, heart's desire, or destiny.

Located in the torso of the body, with the heart chakra at its center, the Human realm draws inspiration from the universal consciousness of the Heaven realm to manifest in the Earth realm. Likewise, through the Human realm, as we ground that inspiration, our day-to-day lives are elevated towards Heaven.

As a Law, *Chi Moves in the Space Between* is the Heavenly component of the Human triad, providing the guidance for this realm. Just as air flows between, among and around trees, mountains and buildings, we can draw the chi of inspiration from the Heaven realm between, among and around any blocks inherent to being humans, that cause us to forget that, in essence, we are each, on a quantum level pure energy, pure Spirit.

The Principle of the Human triad, *Boundaries Dissolve Barriers*, looks at what "space" actually means in your life, in your relationships, and in your own distinctive ways of being. Your boundaries contain the space within which you define who you are and how you express yourself in the world. The clearer you are about this self-knowing, the less you will find yourself barricaded or suppressed by power struggles, defensiveness and alienation. Once freed in this way, you will be able to express yourself in fresh, unimpeded, and limitless ways.

The Practice of the Human triad, *Cultivate Discernment,* provides the tools and exercises to discover what feeds you and what drains you in your life. These distinctions are fundamental to how you experience the spaciousness to feel and be who you really are at your core. This process will ground you in healthy ways to express your truth, experience your own power, and bring your distinctive gifts to the world around you.

CHAPTER 6
The Current of Joy

HUMAN TRIAD
Joy / Love

**Chi Moves in the
Space Between**

Boundaries   Cultivate
Dissolve Barriers   Discernment

Chi Moves in the Space Between
Law of the Human Triad

*Thirty spokes
meet in the hub.
Where the wheel isn't
is where it's useful.*

*Hollowed out
clay makes a pot.
Where the pot's not
is where it's useful.*

*Cut doors and windows
to make a room.
Where the room isn't,
there's room for you.*

*So the profit in what is
is in the use of what isn't.*

—*Tao Te Ching* (as interpreted by Ursula Le Guin)

The second Law of the *Way of Joy*, *Chi Moves in the Space Between*, provides the vision for the Human realm. Here we access universal guidance or the Heavenly aspect in the context of the Human triad—our relationships, our ability to give and receive love, and to live with the limitations of being human. How do we reclaim our power and create the time and space to access our guidance?

Manuel takes a deep breath and then gently closes the door to his office. He walks over to his desk and stands in front of it. The stack of papers demanding his attention has gotten higher since he responded to his boss's summons to her office—his assistant, Alex, must have been here. The phone is blinking, indicating waiting voice mails that he knows are important. The computer displays an unfinished email that will close the deal with an important new customer. He glances at the grocery list that has fallen to the floor. He takes a deep breath, then lets it out with a heavy sigh.

When you let out a heavy sigh during periods of overwhelm, you may assume you have no alternative but to keep plugging along, or give up for a while and face even greater stress later. However, that sigh is your body sending a cue from your unconscious that you need to breathe, to open up inner space. So Manuel does something different.

He turns his chair away from his cluttered desk, toward the wall, and sits down. He looks at the picture hanging there—last year's photograph of him and the kids in the ocean, grinning as they wave snorkels. He grins back, gives a little wave, then closes his eyes. Manuel brings his attention to his breath, and as his focus shifts, he can feel the tension in his shoulders lessen, his body beginning to relax. As he listens to his breath moving in and out, he imagines turning a knob on a radio, lowering the volume both outside and inside his head. As he enters a state of silence, the world outside the office door fades and he opens the door to stillness. Within that stillness, he remembers the feelings of the ocean waves gently moving him. He imagines the rhythm of the water moving in his body, and slowly he feels his heart slow down and open, his joints relax. He floats in the ocean image, feeling the gentle lifting and lowering of his diaphragm as he breathes into the flow of his own life force.

At the conclusion of his meditation, Manuel returns to the tasks at hand, engaged in his work. By the end of the day, he's astonished to see how much he has accomplished in the afternoon and how easily everything seemed to flow.

When Manuel shut his door and turned away from his desk, he took a moment to breathe, shifting his energy away from the stress he was feeling and towards his own inner guidance. He intentionally made a choice to give himself time and space away from the urgency of his tasks. "Taking space," he moved "outside of the box" and entered a different dimension, an elastic moment that stretched out. Seeing the photo of his vacation with his kids stimulated a memory, bringing Manuel back to his heart and away from the brain mutter of the day's demands. These choices provided him with a shift of energy that took him out of a state of discomfort and overwhelm. He was later able to accomplish easily much of what he had to do. We often believe we don't have time to stop and take a moment's break. The paradox is that when we do, time becomes elastic, and we actually feel as though we've ended up with more time.

Much has been written about the health benefits of meditation, particularly in the area of stress reduction. I believe that, on an energetic level, any practices that create an internal opening—whether they be still meditation or automatic writing, moving Chi Kung or prayer—create a sense of *space*, both in the psychological sense of "taking space" and physically inside of the very cells of our bodies, because as we breathe deeply, we oxygenate our blood. We can then open up the energy bound up in stress and transform it into something that can serve us instead of drain us. This is what we do by honoring the "space between."

Heaven within the Human Triad

It has been said that it is the space between the bars that holds the tiger, and it is the silence between the notes that makes the music. It is out of the silence, or the gap, or that space between our thoughts that everything is created, including our own bliss.
— *Wayne Dyer*

Anytime we move outside of the "doingness" of our lives, even for a short suspended moment, we enter into the "gap" or the place "between the notes" where we can connect with our own vitality and a renewed source of energy. When you choose to create this kind of opening in a day, regardless of how you do it, you hold for that moment the key to accessing the Heaven realm. It is in the "space between" that you will hear the wisdom and guidance of Heaven within the Human triad and so enhance the flow of chi.

I believe at any given moment, like Manuel, you actually have the ability to "pivot" energy and create the space that allows the free flow of chi to give direction to your life force. This is essential because expressing your true nature is at the core of the Human triad. When you take time to sit still and breathe, thinking of what you are grateful for or remembering a happy moment, you open space and induce a different energetic vibration, shifting your perception about everything around you. This different perspective, in turn, changes your actual experience.

This shift in perception is then mirrored in surprising ways. For example, have you been in a room full of people when someone walked in with a certain lightness of being, and it seemed as though the energy in the whole room changed? The primary challenge of this Law, *Chi Moves Through the Space Between,* is to intentionally create such openings.

On an energetic level, stress is actually stagnant chi. When things pile up in our lives and in our psyches, we either become exhausted and depressed, or hyper and driven, or some combination. With *Balance Brings Harmony* (the Human Principle of the Heaven triad), I spoke about how crucial it is to anticipate contraction and to open to the space inside of that contraction, in the same way your lungs expand as you inhale. Here, with this Law (the Heaven aspect of the Human triad), you carry forward that lesson. When you can access a sense of spaciousness, regardless of how busy you are, your chi will move freely and bring about transformation.

The Flow of Chi: The Presence in Absence

My first visceral understanding of how *Chi Moves in the Space Between* came when I was learning an elaborate style of *tway shou* (push hands or pushing hands) when I was in my early twenties. As I mentioned earlier, I had the opportunity to study an extended set of push hands with Chinese master, Kwong Ying-Cheng (known in New York at that time as Franklin Y.C. Kwong). A quiet, unassuming man, Dr. Kwong was one of the most precise and powerful teachers I have ever worked with.

Push hands, as I described earlier, is a way to practice the elements of Taiji with a partner. In his book *T'ai Chi*, written with Robert Smith, Tai Chi master Cheng Man-Ch'ing said the aim for the novice practitioner should be to "throw every bone and muscle wide open so that the c'hi may travel unobstructed."[1] Push hands trains practitioners to sense in a very literal way not only the space within their own bodies where chi travels, but also to discover how that unobstructed chi flows in the space between two people.

In the practice, each partner gently tries to push the other off balance, as the other person tries to deflect the push. You learn to sense where there is an open space to direct your chi to unseat your opponent. In turn, in order to deflect your partner's push, you establish and maintain an energetic, chi-filled space around you. This practice of creating space where chi can move requires moving out of a state of *reaction* (where you would either resist or collapse your energy) into one of *response* where you non-defensively maintain your own center.

What struck me most about Dr. Kwong's technique when I pushed hands with him was that his touch was ephemeral, lighter than a down feather, almost as though there was no contact between us at all. When I pushed him, he flowed so easily in the direction I'd initiated I could barely feel him. When he pushed me, it was equally gentle, yet the force of chi moving through an energy field could have easily thrown me off my feet had I not deflected at exactly the right moment.

Quantum Physics and the Space Between

Quantum physicists propose that, on a molecular level, life and all that we consider to be "reality" can be reduced down to space. In essence, that space is, as University of Oregon physics professor, Amit Goswami, Ph.D., puts it, "merely a field of possibilities."[2] Or, as William Tiller, Ph.D., says, "the particles take up an insignificant amount of the void of an atom or molecule ...The rest of it is vacuum."[3]

According to this branch of science, not only do we live inside of space that is an actual energy field, but that space lives inside of us in our very cells and atoms. Deepak Chopra says,

> If you could see the body ...as a physicist could see it, all you'd see is atoms. And if you could see the atoms as they really are, not through the artifact of sensory experience, you'd see these atoms of particles (sic) that are moving at lightning speeds around huge empty spaces. These particles aren't material objects at all. They are fluctuations of energy and information in a huge void of energy and information.... If I could see your body not through this sensory artifact, I'd see a huge empty void with a few scattered dots and a few random electrical discharges here and there. 99.999999% of your body is empty space! And the .000001% of it that appears as matter is also empty space. So, it's all empty space.[4]

This concept, that everything we see as material or solid is ultimately space with "a few random electrical discharges" perceivable by their movement in relationship to one another is hard to even imagine. It's easier to imagine on a macrocosmic level, because we can look through a telescope and see planets with vast amounts of space between them. Even without a telescope, we can see stars suspended in the expanse of the night sky. It is easier to conceptualize "outer space" than "inner space." It's far more difficult to visualize or accept the notion that our bodies are made up of the same space as the universe that we perceive as outside of ourselves.

Yet science is telling us that, on a molecular level, cells are microcosms within a larger energy body, just like the cosmos. In a sense, within each of us is a microscopic universe. Quantum physics thus gives us a context to better understand how chi moves within us, how we can have more power to change our own health when we know how to maximize the movement of that chi. It also challenges our concept of reality by providing data that says *no* form of matter—neither our bodies nor the chair we sit on—is actually solid, but rather is energy moving within a space. This data gives credence to how Chi Kung masters and accomplished martial artists perform seemingly impossible feats.

During a beginning level belt test when I was training in the fighting martial art of Kajukenbo, I was asked to break a solid wooden board with a hand strike. It seemed utterly impossible. Moreover, an acquaintance I'd met a year earlier had broken some bones in her hand trying to do this very thing. Her swollen aching fingers peeking out of a cast were as clear in my mind as the thick board that loomed in front of me. My Sifu, Colleen, who was holding it, smiled reassuringly and affirmed that I could do this, all I needed to do was picture my hand on the other side of the board. But I was so terrified and doubtful I could barely hear her. Although I was awarded my orange belt for succeeding in other elements of the belt test, I was indeed unable to break the board and carried my swollen (though unbroken) wrist and hand around afterwards with no small amount of shame.

Although I was not particularly muscular, I knew the ability to break that board didn't depend my strength, or how much force I applied. Over the next several weeks, I began to think of the board as made up of particles and space, and that my hand, also made up of particles and space, could have the ability to displace those particles through motion. All I needed to do, I told myself, was to travel through the space that was the board. Soon after this image came to me, I was able to break a board in class easily, painlessly, and with some exhilaration. In fact, for me as an early rank martial artist, it became a favorite accomplishment because, given my slight frame, it seemed as though I had turned "reality" inside out, where what was solid became transparent.

At the same time I learned that chi could indeed move through space, even if that space seemed to be solid wood, I also discovered the profound importance of *how* chi gets directed. As long as my focus was on breaking the board, I risked injuring myself. Only when I turned my intention to moving through the *space* of that board could I succeed. This perception was enhanced several years later when an acquaintance told me she had seen Khaleghl Quinn, give a lecture-demonstration during which she broke a board *before* her hand actually made contact with it.

Healing and the Space Between

The understanding that chi moves more effectively through open space than pushing up against a block, is an essential premise in Traditional Chinese Medicine. Dr. Michael Mayer, a psychologist, hypnotherapist and Chi Kung teacher, describes working with a client who had been in an accident. He recounts,

> Terry told me that another health practitioner told her to imagine putting healing energy into the pain in her right leg; but that just made it more swollen. This illustrates the Taoist notion that when there is an excess of yang we want to decrease the energy there, not increase it, as may happen when we concentrate too much on a point that is already suffering from excess. I told her to experiment with focusing, not on the spot that was hurting, but on the "river" above and below that spot...In the first session Terry ... was amazed because this was the most pain-free she had been without medication since her accident six months before... In our second meeting she was able for the first time to experience a zero S.U.D.S. (subjective units of distress) level.[5]

Similarly, when Frank, a middle-aged man, came to my Chi Kung class complaining of his chronically aching hip, I asked him to sit in a comfortable position that neither stretched nor put undue stress on his hips. In the opening meditation of the class, I invited students to focus on a moment in the last day, week, or year where they experienced a feeling of joy. Once they could picture that memory, we began the internal Chi Kung practice called the *Inner Smile*, developed by Mantak Chia, founder of *The Healing Tao*. We allowed the memory of a joyful moment to bring a smile to our faces, then moved the image of that smile to different organs in the body.

At the conclusion of the meditation, Frank was excited to announce that by keeping his attention on moving his smile, the pain in his hip had completely subsided. Like Terry, when Frank brought his attention to directing the movement of chi with his smile, rather than "working out" the pain by trying to stretch it or otherwise focus on it, he was able to release the block.

I think this concept holds profound implications for healing other kinds of trauma—emotional, psychological, and/or spiritual as well. Even when a person makes a conscious, sincere effort to get over a traumatic event, a continued process of only focusing on the event itself may make the pain worse over time, rather than healing it.

Several years ago, a student gave me an article by Dr. Garret Yount, a neuroscientist and brain tumor expert at the California Pacific Medical Center. In 2000, Dr. Yount began a series of experiments to examine the impact of mental intentionality on cancer cells placed on petri dishes. Specifically, he was looking at cell growth rates that were measured before and after Chi Kung healers directed their chi towards those cells.

In one of his earliest articles about this experiment, Dr. Yount wrote:

> The first challenge was to determine the type of intentionality most appropriate for a healer to maintain toward cultured cancer cells isolated from a now deceased patient …a concept that held little meaning to his world view. We came up with two conditions for treating the cancer cells in this experiment. The first one I labeled 'Intent to Kill' because I asked the healer to 'zap the cells with his energy' for twenty minutes and try to kill the cells. The second condition was labeled 'Neutral Intentionality' because the cells were simply placed in front of the healer for twenty minutes while he sat calmly in his meditative state—without 'zapping' and attempting to kill the cells.[6]

Dr. Yount also included a baseline group that received no Chi Kung treatment. After three weeks, all three groups of cells had begun to die, but the neutral group, where the Chi Kung was performed as a general practice without actually directing energy against the cells to kill them, was the one that showed accelerated death. Directing the energy to kill the cells was also successful, but less so than the "neutral" group. Finally, the baseline group, the cells that received no treatment, experienced the least impact. Dr. Yount goes on to say,

> It turned out that the Neutral Intentionality treatment showed the most dramatic effect. The cells died off very rapidly compared to the other treatment group and a group of cells left in a separate room as a control. This surprised me a bit but the healer had predicted it—as a traditional Chinese medical practitioner he aims to balance energies, and he felt that maintaining the 'intent to kill' would interfere with his natural healing field. It appears that he was right.[7]

What struck me most about this experiment is that when the Chi

Kung masters were doing practices that imbued the environment around them with healthy chi rather than directing their chi against the diseased cells to kill them, the cancer cells had the least chance of surviving. Even in the face of an "enemy" like disease, chi moves best when it is expansive and open, even *more* powerful in that state than when directed against a block. Chi moves in the space between just as the roots of a seedling, seeking nourishment, push deep into the earth around sticks, stones and obstacles or water moves around rocks, adapting and flowing.

Journal entry: Want to install a solar light near the entry of my home. I dig a hole in the rocky, impacted ground here in Trinity County, where gold miners, many of them Chinese, built rock-enforced channels to redirect streams of water for their prospecting efforts, I wish for my pick back in Oakland. Want to just Blast Through. I take a deep breath, exhale impatience, then search with the edge of my shovel for the places I can slide in, so pebbles, stones, rocks dislodge themselves. I don't have the strength to break up the rocks anyway—I can only wriggle into the spaces between, let my chi flow to where I sense opening. My shovel carries my chi, the rocks are the block as I try to find the open spaces. Feels like my writing process!

Chi moving in the space between can move us through our own obstacles far more effectively than when we try to force them away. Digging in that rocky soil was much like when I was able to break a board by moving in the space between rather than trying to pit my physical strength *against* it. Although I've had to work to remember it many times in my life, the principle remains true: when we "fight against" barriers to our goals, we are less powerful than when we use a positive flow of energy to create passageways.

The spiritual martial art of Aikido embodies this theory. Aikido founder and sensei, Morihei Ueshiba, has said, "It is important not to be concerned with thoughts of victory and defeat. Rather, you should let the ki of your thoughts and feelings blend with the Universal. Aikido is not an art to fight with enemies and defeat them. It is a way to lead all human beings to live in harmony with each other as though everyone were one family. The secret of Aikido is to make yourself become one with the universe and to go along with its natural movements. One who has attained this secret holds the universe in him/herself and can say, 'I am the universe.'"[8] The world-view of this practice, as I see it, leads us right back to the world of quantum physics.

Empty Space, The Womb of Creation

Our lives can get so caught up in the narratives of what is happening that we can easily forget we are energetic beings made up of the same phenomenon of space and particles as all physical matter. To enter that state of consciousness is to enter a realm that is all-time, all-space. Here is where you receive guidance about how to transform "a field of possibilities" by directing your chi to align with your intention.

Quantum physicists suggest that all of what we consider to be reality is actually formed by how our minds perceive those possibilities, a perception that stems from several factors. In other words, how we form thought influences what we experience. Once again, in that belt test, when I saw that block of wood and perceived only a block, I was unable to break it. When my perception changed, so did my reality; I encountered matter as empty space, and easily broke through the block.

> Deepak Chopra asks,
> The question is what is this empty space? Is it an emptiness of nothing or a fullness of non-material intelligence? In fact it is a fullness of non-material intelligence. ...And with that definition, it's very obvious that this empty space is not an emptiness of nothing but a womb of creation...And nature goes back exactly to that same place, to fashion a galaxy and a rain forest, as it goes to fashion a thought. It's the same place... It's inside us, it's our inner space which gives rise with amazing fertility to all these things that are so crucial to us.[9]

Opening to that "empty space" is not something many of us do easily. When you don't take time to step outside the restrictions of daily demands, you won't be able to quiet your mind. When you don't, some part of you will likely try to slow down or even stop you. For instance, you might hear a rush of voices telling you aren't measuring up, you've totally messed up, or other negating messages—voices that pummel you, blocking your creativity, your ability to follow your heart, and, ultimately, restricting your evolution.

If you give yourself time outside of this inner cacophony, you will give space for your chi to flow and in so doing, open the portal to hear the Source of universal wisdom and to your own strength.

As so many spiritual traditions teach, meditation and/or prayer can bring us back to a mindful, intentional connection to that opening. In her interpretation of the fifteenth hexagram of the I Ching, "Modesty," Ma Deva Padma writes, "Simplicity creates spaciousness; whether we are clearing unnecessary clutter from a room or from our minds, the result is not only refreshing and expansive, but a new perspective is gained as well."[10]

When we avoid spending time in the stillness of inner space, we don't have access to the universal pool of consciousness, and we lose many chances to have spontaneous, transforming insights. While I don't "blame" people who suffer from illness for causing it, I do believe that blocks to our own healing can become bigger over time if we don't resolve them, causing physical symptoms.

A minister told me a story about a young man who came to her for counsel. He wanted to reconcile his spirituality with his sexuality. Initially, he presented this question merely as an exploration, saying he wasn't really sure where he was going to go with it. He had been raised in a fairly fundamentalist sect and although he had moved away from those beliefs, he still wasn't quite sure how to integrate his spiritual practice and his sexuality.

This minister told me that one day, after they had been talking for months about his choices and his yearnings, he came in and said, "I'm really out of it today because I have this horrible ear infection. I've been through three courses of antibiotics and I just can't get rid of it. I can barely hear; my ears are just so clogged." He felt scared because the prescribed antibiotics weren't working and the doctor was saying surgery, or some other kind of invasive procedure, might be necessary.

The young man was a college student and was very stressed because he was missing classes. The minister decided talking was not particularly useful at that point—and asked him if he'd be open to receiving some Reiki.

After his treatment, she had him turn over on his side with the infected ear down. She placed one hand under his head, over that ear, and the other hand lightly covering his other ear. She stayed quiet for a while and then asked, "Is there anything you're afraid to hear and would you be willing to tell me about it?'"

He suddenly blurted out in a rush of words that he was afraid that his dad would disown him if he told him about his sexuality, that his mother would wish she had never birthed him, and that the Divine would say, "You are no longer Beloved."

The minister continued, "At the moment he said that, liquid started pouring out of his ear, squishing through my fingers. He began to weep, and he wept a long time. I just kept his head in my hands. It was gruesome on one level, but very powerful. I asked him to turn over and liquid drained out of his left ear as well. In three days, his infection was completely gone. Because he hadn't given himself the space to acknowledge what he was most afraid to hear, his ears had literally stopped up."

She concluded her account saying she was able to officiate at his Holy Union with a man a couple of years later. Although his parents weren't able to attend, they sent a down payment on a condo and embraced him and his male partner.

When you move out of a state of mind-chatter that is inundated by negating or punitive voices, you can enter that quiet space, set apart. Then you can recognize voices from the past that you've outgrown, or voices from the present that undermine your strength. When you breathe into space and listen inside, you'll discern which messages are helpful and which are not. When your chi moves freely, your heart will open and the blocks that have obstructed you will no longer stop you from healing and moving forward on your life's path.

Sometimes within that space you will find deeply transformative information, the inspiration that makes you change a life course. But the Heaven Law of *Chi Moves through Space Between* can be useful in our Human realm, our day-to-day challenges as well.

A couple of days after a particularly full weekend, during which I'd taught some classes and led a memorial service for a dear friend, I decided to take a short walk to a creek near my house. Normally this act would recharge me—walking in Nature, listening to the sounds of the creek and wind in the trees, practicing Chi Kung at the water's edge. Indeed, when I was at the creek feeling a little better, I decided to take a longer loop to get home. A few minutes after I left the creek-side, I was hit with a level of fatigue beyond what I could have anticipated. I felt as though I could hardly stand up, let alone walk for another hour or so. As I was going up a little hill, I was suddenly stopped by the thought, "This isn't working, I don't feel good, and this isn't helping me. Not only that, I don't think I can make it home. What," I asked myself, "would replenish me?"

As I stood thinking, looking down at the path in front of me, a gentle voice seemed to say "Just lie down on this path, where your feet have so often walked. Here you will ground." It was raining and my rational mind argued, "No, get home before you're too wet and get sick." With some deep breaths, my body made my decision for me. Sinking down to the ground, I rolled onto my back, feeling the raindrops on my face. It was a deeply comforting release as I lay there with the support of the sweet-smelling dirt below me. I drifted. As I did, I remembered that Khaleghl had once told me that her Cherokee grandmother had taught her that one way to replenish your energy when you are drained is to lie on your back on the ground. Once recharged, I walked home understanding that I had finally opened space inside of the contraction that followed my big energetic output of the previous weekend.

Conclusion: Infinity in the Space Between

It has been said that it is through the heart, the center of the Human realm, that we may discover the portal to the detached compassion that characterizes Spirit...In the traditions, Spirit is found neither in Heaven nor in Earth, but in the heart. The Heart has always been seen as the integration or the union point of Heaven and Earth, the point that Earth grounded Heaven and Heaven exalted Earth. Neither Heaven nor Earth alone could capture Spirit; only the balance of the two found in the Heart could lead to the secret door beyond death and mortality and pain.
— Ken Wilber

As the Heaven aspect of the Human triad, the Law *Chi Moves in the Space Between* teaches us that all is ultimately space, whether perceived through the vast macrocosm of the cosmos, or the microcosmic space within our cells and everything around us. Unobstructed energy moves through this space, this "gap," as freely and abundantly as currents of air, water, blood, or electricity.

When you discover the space around you and inside of you where your chi runs freely, you will find your way back to your heart. As Ken Wilber says "the Heart has always been seen as the integration or the union point of Heaven and Earth."[11] Through your heart, center of the Human realm, you bring the inspiration of Heaven to the manifestation of Earth. At the same time, you expand your awareness that all that appears to be material and Earthbound is, in its very essence, the same as the intangible infinity of Heaven.

CHAPTER 7
The Vessel of Joy

HUMAN TRIAD
Joy / Love

Chi Moves in the
Space Between

Boundaries   Cultivate
Dissolve Barriers   Discernment

Boundaries Dissolve Barriers
Principle of the Human Triad

I believe it is through our vulnerability that we experience our greatest power.
— *Sharon Strand Ellison*

As the Principle of the Human triad, *Boundaries Dissolve Barriers* draws from the perspective of this triad's Heavenly Law, *Chi Moves in the Space Between,* and looks at how you might be inspired to apply the information from the Law in ways applicable to your own life. How do you create "space" so that your energy flows in how you make choices, interact in relationships, and achieve goals?

Because the Human triad is at the center of the three triads, this Principle, at the center of the triad, becomes the center of the entire set of nine Laws, Principles and Practices that make up the whole *Way of Joy* system. Since the Human realm is about how we use our heart, motivated by joy, to create our individual expression, it means that how we create boundaries is an essential tool for the fulfillment in following our heart's path.

As the second Principle of the *Way of Joy, Boundaries Dissolves Barriers* follows from the previous Principle from the Heaven triad, *Balance Brings Harmony.* The story that follows shows how these two Principles interrelate.

A Harmonic Boundary

If the body can respond so decisively to music, it must in some sense be music.
— Don G. Campbell

Several years ago I was invited to teach Chi Kung in a workshop for singers taught by the improvisational jazz singer, Rhiannon. During one session, Rhiannon divided everyone into two groups to practice harmonizing. At one point in the exercise, the two groups had to sing a "second," a very difficult chord to sing in tune because the two notes are so close together. The singers found themselves sliding from the note they were supposed to be singing to the note right next to it, which the other group was singing. They practiced the chord again and again trying to stay on key, but simply couldn't do it. It was too difficult to hear the other group's note without losing their own.

After witnessing a certain amount of struggle, I offered to teach them a Chi Kung exercise called *Pebble in the Lake*, (p. 156) which works with establishing energetic boundaries. This form develops your awareness of both what is happening inside of you and what is happening in the environment around you as well as your ability to hold awareness of the two simultaneously. In the form, you draw your energy into a small ball of chi with your hands. This ball, like the Tao symbol, contains your wholeness, the balance of what you perceive both internally and externally. Once you gather your awareness into this concentrated whole, you drop that ball down into the "lake" of your pelvis, creating a ripple effect in that energy field so that it moves out from your center into wider and wider concentric circles that form an energetic boundary.

I asked them to practice the chord together while doing the exercise. They were able to do it on the first try! After they practiced the Chi Kung a little longer, where they established a field of simultaneous awareness (where they could hear both their own note and the other), I asked them to take a deep breath, relax, and imagine the field of energy they created as they sang. The harmony held true and they were able to continue the song in good spirits.

In the chapter *Balance Brings Harmony*, I defined harmony as the ability to experience more than one note at the same time. There, we looked at how this correlates to our ability to balance different levels of awareness, to experience the interdependence of opposites, and so on. Containing difference, even opposition, in our lives or our psyches without dismissing any single aspect is the means with which we can balance the universal vision of the Heaven realm with the day-to-day reality of the Earth realm.

In *Boundaries Dissolve Barriers,* we learn how our boundaries contain and hold that balance. As the singers discovered when they practiced *Pebble in the Lake,* in order to stay true to the purity of their own note while being able to hear and harmonize with a different note, they needed to create and hold a literal energetic boundary.

Barriers: A World Without Boundaries

We are constantly in communication with everything around us...a kind of conscious electricity that transmits and receives message to and from other people's bodies.
— *Caroline Myss*

When two people meet and each one is in an open, expansive place, they are likely to have a meeting not only of minds, but of hearts and souls as well. On the other hand, if one feels the other "takes up too much space" or there is "just not enough room for me," then that person is likely to construct a barrier to keep the other person out. The person may construct the barrier internally by being withholding or insincere, or externally by becoming judgmental or aggressive, or by withdrawing.

I believe we create barriers as a block to protect ourselves when we don't have boundaries. Barriers are a psychic "keep out" sign erected to hold others at a distance when we feel at risk. I think we most often lose our sense of self when we're with someone who is invasive or demanding and/or because we show caring in ways that are co-dependent, causing us to merge with the other. In either case, when we are afraid we'll give away more than feels right, our internal response tends to become antagonistic. Our thoughts, feelings, or actions focus on keeping the other at a distance.

The Nature of Barriers

Random House Dictionary defines barriers as a) anything built or serving to bar passage; b) any natural bar or obstacle (mountain); c) anything that restrains or obstructs progress or access; d) an Antarctic ice shelf. These words, *bar, restrain, obstruct,* all imply some kind of block.

In our own lives, we create barriers as a way to make some part of ourselves inaccessible to others especially when we feel vulnerable, afraid, alienated, or even when we simply want to avoid a situation we think might be unpleasant. We erect these blocks to protect ourselves yet such barriers even when done passively or indirectly are an adversarial attempt to create boundaries.

Have you ever found yourself in a meeting where a facilitator looks directly at you, expecting some kind of response, but you didn't want to be the one to give it? Or, have you been in a group of people being selected for a team, and you didn't want to be picked? Did you look away, try to make yourself smaller, refuse to make eye contact? Or, perhaps, you stared at the person defiantly with a "don't you dare" look. In any of these situations, you were putting up a barrier.

Once we've established a barrier, we often go out of our way to keep it intact. For instance, Susan goes to the supermarket to buy some broccoli. As she approaches the produce section, she sees Mark, her best friend's ex-boyfriend (the Cad), picking out some onions. As he turns towards the greens, their eyes meet briefly. Susan darts over to the dog food aisle even though she doesn't have a pet. She pretends to pore over the labels on cans of Alpo until she sees Mark leave the store. Here, Susan is hiding behind the literal barrier of a supermarket aisle because she's afraid that if she so much as says 'hello,' she'll be caught in a conversation where she feels like she has to pretend to be friendly. She doesn't trust herself to have an adequate boundary. There are countless ways we might create barriers every day—from not returning a phone call to lying about our plans to hiding behind a book or TV screen.

Ironically, I think we also erect barriers even when we feel overly merged with another person. For example, John and Linda fell in love. They spent as much time together as possible. They became so close, they could finish each other's sentences. An expectation grew between them that they would always agree.

But every now and then, feeling the need for some space, Linda would lash out or push John away. Sensitive and not knowing what to do, John would feel betrayed and retreat into his own sulk. Because neither one could feel where she or he left off and the other began, tension grew and barriers sprang up. For both of them, a sense of alienation escalated. One evening, for example, when John asked Linda what she'd like for dinner, she avoided expressing her preference in an attempt to stay connected. Later, while they were talking about weekend plans, she mentioned that she was planning to have breakfast with Mary, and John said, "Oh, I thought we'd go to the Farmer's Market together." Feeling inexplicably trapped, she yelled, "I can spend time with a friend if I want to. We don't have to do *everything* together."

Over time, John felt betrayed, as though Linda had turned out to be the opposite of the person he'd once been so close to. He felt he couldn't trust his own perceptions anymore. Linda felt as though she had suppressed her needs, lost her freedom and sense of individuality. Both felt that they had in some way sacrificed their sense of self. They finally separated.

In the end, I believe creating barriers is never as safe or effective as having good boundaries because barriers include in their very nature a need to block others and to defend self. That need to defend implies a lack of either self-definition or some lack of security in protecting one's own space. I think barriers occur when we are concerned we will not be able to be or act as we want, whether because of our own choices or because of someone else's power over us. The impact this has both on our own self-esteem and on our relationships is profoundly erosive.

I've been in situations not unlike that of John and Linda. A lack of boundaries, a tendency to merge, has always been one of my most difficult personal issues. As a rule, I think I've tended to over-identify with others and forget myself. This leads to feeling either as though I have to control them, to be somehow responsible for what they say or think, or the reverse, where I forget I might see things differently. In either scenario, I end up feeling as though I'm outside of myself, and must erect some kind of barrier to disentangle my identity from the other.

We do not set up barriers only in relationship to others. How often have you found yourself in a state of resistance, in which you have blocked off your own internal process? When we construct these barriers, we impede our creativity, not permitting it to flow in a specific direction. While barriers block our inspiration and our ability to follow through, boundaries actually give shape to our creative impulses.

From Barriers to Boundaries

What would it mean to set a healthy boundary instead of erecting barriers? How can we experience a sense of our self without becoming rigid and hard?

In Chinese medicine, *wei chi* has been described as the body's first line of defense against infection, germs or disease. Analogously, in Chi Kung, *wei chi* simply signifies protective energy. It's a protection that comes from being open, expansive, and assertive. It originates from a place of "I am" as opposed to "you can't." Protection, in this case, doesn't mean being able to defend yourself. Instead, it is the ability to exude so much radiant energy or *chi* that nothing negative can penetrate it. It's as though you are so surrounded by the positive that the negative or draining becomes irrelevant.

I have found the idea of using an open, expansive energy as a kind of protection, even from physical danger, is foreign to most people. More often, people think that to protect themselves they need to block negative energy, whether from a physical or emotional attack. I first decided to study martial arts so that I could feel safer on the streets. By the time I was in my late twenties, I had had several street attack experiences, two of which involved a man grabbing my breast.

The first incident occurred in New York City when I was about nineteen. I had been studying Aikido for about six months and loved both the philosophy and the acrobatics of the art. I felt efficient, even cocky, in the way only students in their early days of training can feel.

I was walking down a street in Manhattan one day, my mind drifting, when a man approached me from the opposite direction. As he was passing, he shot out a hand and quickly squeezed my left breast. Before I realized what had happened, it was over and he had disappeared around the corner. I was devastated and afraid. But most of all I was disappointed in myself, chagrined that I had not come up with some brilliant twist, turn and throw that would have protected me and landed him on his butt.

My second experience happened in Paris about six years later. I was standing on a street corner talking to my boyfriend, oblivious to who was around me, when I felt a sharp tightening on my breast. I looked down in time to see a hand releasing me. As the man strode by, he called out an insolent "merci" to my boyfriend, who stood gaping after him.

Not long after that incident I returned to the States, moved to California, and subsequently began to study Kajukenbo to learn self-defense. It wasn't until six years later, when I was in my mid-thirties, that I had my first conscious experience of *wei chi*.

"I'm sick of fighting. I'm tired of punching, kicking, hitting. There has to be some other way."

Lost in my thoughts, I trudge home from BART after a long workout at the kwoon[1]. I can feel myself sagging as Mission Street swirls around me, heightening its end-of-the-day frenzy. My shoulders hunch, my spine droops and I catch myself muttering out loud, "It's got to stop." Shaking myself aware, I look up and notice a guy approaching from half a block away. I recognize the attitude, the swaggering stride, even though I've never seen him before. Near-sighted, I can't really make out his features, but I can feel in my skin how his lips curl slightly as he spots me.

"No," I think calmly, walking taller. My spine unfurls as the top of my head lifts up towards the sky. I take a deep breath and relax as he gets near. 'I am here. I am me.' He reaches out his hand to grab when a "frisson," a shivery sensation, spirals up my back. I look down to see his hand bounce away an inch or two from

contact with my breast. No contact. It is as though he has hit a bubble of air, of resilience, trampolining back away from me. We pass one another. I turn my head to look back at him. His face, turned towards me, has an expression that is a mixture of both incredulity and fear. Slowly, he looks down at his hand, still clawed open to grab, then back up at me, back down, then up. He takes a few backward steps, then turns and hurries away, swagger-less.

In a moment of synchronicity, I protected myself without needing to make physical contact just when I was thinking about my dissatisfaction with external fighting forms. This was a pivot point that sparked a life change for me. Excited, if mystified, by what had happened, I returned home to find a telephone message from Khaleghl Quinn, a new friend and colleague I'd recently met while we were both teaching at a martial arts camp in Holland. In yet another moment of synchronicity, Khaleghl's message included some of her thoughts about ways I might work with my chi outside of the context of the martial art I was practicing. I decided to stop training in Kajukenbo and begin a weekly commute to Santa Cruz to study Chi Kung with her. Not long after, I learned that the name for the energetic transmission I'd experienced on Mission Street that day was *wei chi.*

The study of *wei chi,* of protection that is open, expansive, and radiant, is what informs this Principle, *Boundaries Dissolve Barriers.* As I have continued to explore *wei chi* over the years, I've developed a new understanding about boundaries in physical, psychological, and even spiritual landscapes.

The word *boundary* is a way to define or describe space. If we think of our bodies as a temple—a concept common to many spiritual traditions—then the boundaries could be the walls of that temple. They define the space inside. Just as the walls of a room define the shape of its space, boundaries define the shape of our internal space: what we believe/don't believe, think/don't think, or feel/don't feel. As we saw with the Law of this triad, *Chi Moves in the Space Between,* on a purely physical plane, that space itself, what we are made of—cells, atoms, quarks, energetic particles—is the same in all life forms, all matter. It is the external shape those particles within space take that defines us, makes us perceivable.

I believe that the wisdom of and access to the shape of our internal space resides in our bodies. For instance, when have you just had a "gut feeling" about something, or been in a complex situation but have just "known in your heart what was right," or been able to picture something in your "mind's eye"?

An easy way to understand one aspect of your boundaries would be to consider what you absolutely know to be true for yourself. For example, if I say, "I love lasagna," or "I have no desire to learn carpentry," these things are part of who I am. No one can tell me that actually I hate lasagna, or that I've always wanted to work with wood. And even though I might consider arguments saying lasagna might not be healthy to eat every day, or that I would be a more self-sufficient woman if I knew carpentry, it is still up to me to know what I want to do with that information. It is part of my self-definition, my boundary. I can make different choices in relation to that boundary, but the inner truth of it remains constant.

I suggest that our boundaries describe a space that is ours: our own particular thoughts, values, feelings and actions.[2] I believe that we create boundaries for each aspect of our being—physical, emotional, mental and spiritual and that these boundaries in turn shape our individuality.

As I mentioned earlier, boundaries also play an essential role in how we express our creativity. In fact, as most artists would acknowledge, setting limits is essential to the shaping of any successful piece. Limits, in this case, are freeing. They provide a structure in which the inspiration for spontaneous expression can occur. When an artist, be it a choreographer, writer, or composer, is asked to "just create" and does not have some kind of internal structure or limits, the task becomes too overwhelming. A choreographer, for example, might play with levels—high/low, or dynamics—slow/ fast, or texture of movement—hard/soft. A playwright might choose a time, place and certain characters to create a piece. A novelist might concentrate on an era, an environment and the arc of a story. A musician might choose a theme, melody or rhythm to explore.

The creative impulse comes from the Heaven realm. It remains ethereal and in a state of potential until, in the Human realm, we give it boundaries to shape it. Without a structure of some kind, the expression of inspiration loses its ability to build on itself and dies out with a sense of there being either too much or too little to say. Expression becomes chaotic, meaningless.

Our boundaries define our individuality, empower us to fulfill our creative impulses and give expression to our uniqueness. At the same time, I believe boundaries are not only the ways we distinguish ourselves from one another, but are also the means through which we touch one another. Where one person's boundaries intersect or overlap with another's is the point at which the two can meet with open minds and hearts, the qualities missing in the "barriered" example at the beginning of this chapter. In this sense, boundaries both separate and connect us.

Boundaries and Barriers in My Own Life

My father disowned me for the first time when, at age 18, I told him I was going to live with my boyfriend. His reaction astounded me even though he had never been a particularly active parent when I was growing up. A remote presence even though he worked at home, I felt a special bond with him, stemming from treasured memories such as when he'd invite me into his study when I was in second grade (and younger), play a melodic passage from an orchestral piece he was working on, then pause and ask me, "So, whaddya think, Vic? D'ya like it?" Or the many moments of vital connection I felt when I danced to his music, music that I also awoke to every morning. So, naively, I was shocked by his reaction to my news; the subsequent rift lasted 10 years.

Many years after the end of that first relationship, when I was living in San Francisco, my father and I began to tentatively reconnect once again—until he discovered I was a lesbian. A new period of dissolution began. Letters flew back and forth between us. His were condemning and angry while mine ranged from plaintively self-righteous, "Why can't you just love me as I am, unconditionally!?" to defiant, "Well, I'm happy and I like who I am." His final letter to me ended with the words "since you like who you are and I don't, I think it would be best if we not see one another anymore."

After that, I did sometimes write notes to him when I heard he had been seriously ill or after I was hit by the car. I never heard anything back, although his wife sometimes sent a note she signed for them both.

As years went by and the silence between my father and me congealed, I worked to convince myself that it was OK and to "get on" with my life without thinking too much about him. Sometimes I made light of it, saying he was an Italian patriarch whose daughter could only be a virgin or a mother, with nothing happening in-between with either sex. But I always felt out of integrity, trapped within my own barriers.

Then a chance meeting changed the course of my life. I found myself in a workshop with author Sharon Ellison, the creator of *Powerful Non-Defensive Communication,* a profoundly life-altering process.[3] Sharon's analysis of how our defensiveness arises from using tools of communication based on the rules of war and her alternative process for using these tools in a way that is direct, vulnerable and empowered made absolute sense to me. I made an immediate connection with the concepts I had been teaching about *wei chi* and my thoughts about how boundaries could dissolve barriers. I began to work intensively with Sharon, bringing her to my school for workshops, co-offering retreats, and working privately with her on my own. It was not long before we became close friends.

I talked to Sharon about my relationship with my father, and she suggested writing him a letter using the non-defensive process. In draft after draft, Sharon helped me recognize the different ways I was still being defensive. A year later, I finally sent him my letter, which closed with this limit: "I've tried to imagine your response to this letter and I can't. If you want to write or call, I would probably be amazed as well as happy. I would love to begin a correspondence with you. If you are not willing to write to me, talk to me or see me, or if you respond solely in anger, then I will do my best to let go of having your rejection continue to have power in my life.… Regardless of the outcome, I want you to know I will always love you."

For the first time in many years, I received an immediate reply. His tone was still accusatory, and my initial reaction was to run to Sharon, saying, "See, he *is* impossible!" But she pointed out the ways he was actually simply naming his own view, albeit defensively, and worked with me on my next response. Not long after, I went to see him for the first time in more than 10 years. Over the next eleven years until the end of his life, my relationship with him became clearer, and understanding between us slowly deepened.

In my letter to my father, I held my boundaries in two ways: the first was in how I spoke about what I thought and felt in a complete, vulnerable, yet honest and direct way, and the second by the limit I set. That boundary was the path to creating a deepening intimacy with my father, ultimately dissolving long-held barriers, so that our minds and hearts could finally meet again as they had so many years ago when I danced to his music.

Defining Ourselves from the Inside Out

How clear we are about what we know inside to be right for *us*—as opposed to a strong opinion about others (judgment) or adopting their beliefs about us (merging)—is one part of the intricate structure that creates our boundaries. Clear boundaries allow us to *be* who we are and others to *see* who we are. Another part is to know our strengths and weaknesses. Not expecting to be all things to all people, including ourselves, allows us to claim our own individuality. When we do, openly and non-defensively, we are also able to establish our interdependence, whether in our one-to-one relationships, in our neighborhoods, or in the larger global community.

When we are in truly interdependent (as opposed to independent or co-dependent) relationships, we can further support, strengthen, and relax inside of our own boundaries and, in turn, better accept others' strengths and weaknesses. Without expecting perfection, we can trust the reciprocity in such relationships. In fact, I think the most profound reciprocity comes with this kind of understanding and provides the foundation for gradual transformation. I believe it is only when we are in a clear relationship with ourselves that we can truly feel an authentic intimacy with others.

Boundaries and Spirituality

Boundaries are tools we use to craft our being. On a purely physical plane, our bodies themselves constitute our boundary, with the skin surrounding all the matter that is our physical reality, the matter and the space through which chi moves. On an emotional level, boundaries are the means through which we create reciprocity and intimacy with others. On the level of intellect, boundaries give direction to our creative potential. I also believe that boundaries have a function in the realm of spirituality, how we experience our connection to guidance of the Heaven realm. Whether in a religious or spiritual context or not, I think that many people have a deep desire to connect with a larger perspective, an understanding of something greater than self, whether *or not* it is conceived of as Divine, God(s), Goddess(es), or Higher Power.

Boundaries are the means by which we question, define or experience our personal connection to higher consciousness. After all, spirituality is a purely personal experience. Yet, the experience of connectedness goes beyond any particular spiritual practice. And it is the interrelationship of those two places, internal and external, that constitutes a boundary. I would like to explore three categories as they relate to a relationship with the Divine.

1. Individual Connection

When I was hit by that car in 1990 and experienced myself as a conscious seed living inside of the hull of my body, I experienced a wake-up call that brought me back to Source. This experience has impacted my choices from that moment on and has given me a whole new perspective on life. Some people experience a form of kundalini or awakening, where a sense of enlightenment happens suddenly and dramatically; others can have a less intense experience, one they not might think of as spiritual at all. For example, shortly after a dear, long-time friend of hers died, my mother, who is Jewish but a self-described agnostic, sat alone in the sanctuary of the Presbyterian church where her office was located. As she reflected on his life and their relationship, she felt filled with a sense of quiet peace, as though a comforting presence sat with her. For that moment, I would say that she felt connected to a larger Self.

In her grief, my mother established a boundary, taking time and space away from a busy day at the office, to sit quietly, breathe, pay attention, and so experienced a deep connection with her own individual sense of Spirit. Had she refused to take the time to create that boundary, she would not have made the connection.

2. Self Reflected as Divine

The opportunity to see oneself reflected in a positive light by someone else is, I believe, often what draws people to one another—the experience of being seen and heard for who we "really are." In this sense, we might feel larger than our shortcomings, that our best or highest self has been seen. I think this is what people mean when they say with a sense of relief, "At last I've found someone who really gets who I am."

Have you ever felt, in the throes of an attraction, romantic or intellectual, a sense of power, even omnipotence, clarity and strength, directly associated with how you've seen yourself reflected in someone else's gaze? That sense of feeling larger than life is the second way I think many people experience being god-like.

When we experience our strengths reflected through another's appreciation and acknowledgment, boundaries—knowing both our own limits and strengths—are essential to maintain perspective. Otherwise we are left with trying to live up to some inflated ideal that may not be integrated with our human fallibility, and may actually become harmful because we no longer accept the aspects of self that don't fit that reflection.

3. Divine Through Others

I also believe we experience divinity in the context of boundaries when we find another person—teacher, spiritual leader, or intimate companion—who appears to provide some kind of link to Spirit in their very being. When we are with that person, things fall into place, seem part of a greater plan. A person may say the right thing at the right time so that we are thrust into a greater perspective, almost as though we are looking down at a situation from a higher place. Or, a spiritual leader, whose message reaches the hearts of many, may convey a sense of divine connection to his or her followers. I remember one friend who told me she felt like she was in the presence of God when she was with a certain spiritual teacher. The experience of finding the Divine through others can also occur through the synergy of many people worshipping together.

When we perceive the divine through others, it is crucial that we hold a boundary that keeps us from collapsing into that other, releasing all responsibility for our own spiritual identity and our own powers of discernment. I believe this is what makes the difference between a sycophant and someone on their own spiritual path who finds genuine value in a teacher. While we can certainly be inspired and taught by others, or feel exalted in a community of like-minded people, we each must still be able to discern what is right and wrong for ourselves. My friend who said she felt the presence of God when she was with her teacher later discovered he was sexually and violently abusing several of his female followers. At that point she realized she had become enmeshed in a cult that was life-threatening to herself and others.

Conclusion: An Invitation to Self-Esteem

You are in the truest sense either a human being having an occasional spiritual experience or an infinite spiritual being having a temporary human experience.
— *Wayne Dyer*

In Spirit, we are limitless space—we exist in infinity. As individual beings, our boundaries give shape to the expression of Spirit. I think that in order to have good boundaries, I need to tend to my own temple, cultivate that inner sanctuary, consider who I am as sacred and worth attention. This is an invitation to self-esteem. If we understand Spirit as connection to all-that-is, and perceive we are literally made up of the same particulate matter and space as everything in our environment, we realize our boundaries are the container of that elusive substance. Our body is the vessel that makes us individuals, gives each of us a different face, a different perspective, gives us the gift of distinction. To experience the two together is to experience the "we are all one" consciousness at the same time that we discover and celebrate the richness of our diversity.

We tend to think of boundaries as separating us. However, when our boundaries are not intact, we either co-dependently merge identities or we stand apart, alienated. In both cases we miss the sense of true connection. Ironically it is actually our boundaries that provide the doorway to connection where we can feel both autonomous and where it is that we overlap or meet. When they are intact, we feel more connected to others because we are standing in connection to ourselves.

If I were to distinguish boundaries and barriers as I see them in terms of texture, I'd say boundaries have a quality of flexibility, resilience and strength, like a protective skin or membrane, while barriers are rigid, brittle, or even spiky like a porcupine's quills.

While boundaries define self from the inside out, I think barriers defend self from the outside in. Both are concerned with what we experience inside of ourselves as related to what is happening externally. The more we are able to clearly define ourselves (I believe/don't believe, think/don't think, feel/don't feel, am/am not, will/will not), the less we feel the need to keep guarded or defended in our interactions with others. As a result, barriers simply dissolve.

This is also true when we experience barriers in our own creative process. I have seen my own barriers transform into boundaries during the course of writing this book. When overwhelmed with the task of articulating a difficult concept, my mind seemed to hit that Antarctic ice shelf, the barrier. Instead of trying to push past my writing block, I set a boundary and stopped. This created the space I needed to see how I could transform the stress I was experiencing. So I would weed in my garden until I was able to focus on the one small piece I wanted to address, or I would succumb to a nap and let my unconscious take over.

For my barriers to dissolve, I needed to create a boundary. Boundaries make up the vessel that contains the flow of *Chi in the Space Between*, so I needed to go to where there was a sense of openness, movement, a reconnection with Self. So many times I have seen myself and others become slaves to "should," losing touch with where our joy might be and how it might fuel us in the very direction we fear we are abandoning. The magic of the boundary is that it can free us, provide a way to both rest and move forward in the same or a new direction, and so bring us back to our heart, our Joy's home.

CHAPTER 8
The Choice of Joy

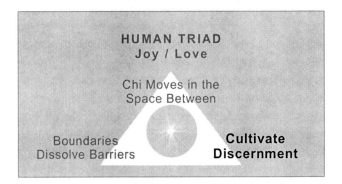

HUMAN TRIAD
Joy / Love

Chi Moves in the
Space Between

Boundaries   **Cultivate**
Dissolve Barriers   **Discernment**

Cultivate Discernment
Practice of the Human Triad

Experience is not what happens to a man;
it is what a man does with what happens to him.
— *Aldous Huxley*

As a young person, Carla was always confident, fully alive. An honor student, she loved to dance, play the guitar and sing. She was often the life of the party and always compassionate toward others. As a young adult, she studied music in college and played in a local band until a critical professor told her she wasn't "talented" enough to "do anything" with her music. While she hadn't made up her mind for sure, she was seriously considering a music career, and the harshly presented criticism devastated her.

After she graduated, she became involved with someone who was also very critical. Her parents had always been extremely supportive, and while she was somewhat conscious of how unsupportive this relationship was compared to her family, Carla assumed that since she was an "adult" now, she couldn't expect things to always be "happy." After being together for three years, she found out her partner was having an affair, and once again she felt devastated and lost.

The trauma of this loss was further compounded by several other losses. She had left her job to move with her partner to a different city and hadn't yet found another job when they separated. Then her grandmother, with whom she was very close, died unexpectedly.

In despair, Carla felt as though she had somehow lost the person she used to be. She felt "fundamentally flawed." When I met her, years later, she told me, "I had an unrelenting negative projection that I was worthless, as though I had no place on the planet. Even when I walked into a grocery store and someone looked at me, I believed people were thinking negative things about me, like I didn't belong there."

Carla moved into a cabin in the mountains outside of Napa Valley and worked at odd jobs to support herself. Although her home was situated in a beautiful natural environment in the redwoods, she felt isolated since she spent most of her time alone.

Carla still played her guitar and sang, finding solace in her music. She began taping herself and playing her music back on her boom box. Her voice sounded grotesque to her, and her body would physically hurt when she heard it. Every time she listened to herself she relived the professor's criticism, only now it came from within. At the time, she didn't understand why she had a compulsion to continue taping herself when the process had become so painful.

Listening to a replay, Carla later told me, "I was feeling that customary cringe of self-judgment. But there was one moment, one note that sounded true. When I heard that authentic note, I had a moment of suspension where—for that instant—I was not in pain. An inner voice said, 'Carla, take this moment and expand on it.' It was like seeing a ray of light in the sky. Something opened, and for that instant I sensed there was a potential for growth."

Carla recognized that soft subtle voice as different from her internalized judgment. She heard it as one of gentle guidance and knew she could expand upon that moment. "This was a pivotal point," she said, "because, from that moment on, whenever I found myself in the pain of self-judgment, I had a tool to deal with it. I'd just suspend all my thoughts and listen. I began to hear or feel that voice consistently. Not a voice exactly, but a gentle impetus. I might be browsing in a bookstore and feel an impulse to buy a certain book, which would turn out to contain something that gave me more tools to work out of the pain I was in.

"It took me some more years to realize it wasn't about how much musical talent I had, or whether I was too flawed to hold onto a man. It was about how I allowed the way others treated me to alter my own view of myself. That note I heard was my own pure creative potential that no one could take away from me. This knowledge became a foundation on which I slowly regained my confidence and love of life."

Holding Discernment in Times of Despair

Wherever you are is the entry point.
— *Kabir*

In this story, Carla was being bombarded by her own self-criticism and negative judgment that had grown out of a series of painful episodes. The optimism and self-confidence she had possessed as a young person had been stripped away.

At the same time, I believe Carla held onto a vital piece of her capacity to discern what she needed: she kept playing her music in spite of the suffering she experienced. Like the sun shining, but hidden behind dark clouds, the pulse of her joy was still somewhere deep within in her music, sustaining her.

Carla's story is a perfect example of the idea expressed by Kabir, that our "entry point" is wherever we are. Her connection to inspiration from the Heaven realm did not exist only when she was confident and strong. Even within a state of deep depression, because of her choice (Human) to keep playing (Earth), she stayed open to her source of inspiration (Heaven).

In the Human triad, *Cultivate Discernment* is ultimately about what choices you make and how you make them. In order to live in alignment with your joy you need to hold the *intention* to make healthy choices that support it. Although not completely aware of it at the time, Carla instinctively followed that path.

The Pivot: Steps in Reconnecting To Source

If the doors of perception were cleansed, everything would appear as it is.
— *William Blake*

It was that *choice* to continue playing and singing—through the clouds of despair—that gave Carla the key to pivot her experience. At the moment of entry, just prior to hearing that "one true note," she lacked awareness of her connection to inspiration; she was at the *point of entry* without knowing it.

When she heard the note, during that "moment of suspension" where she felt no pain and remembered her potential, she moved into the Heaven triad. The guiding voice she heard was the Observer Self, born out of *Stillness in Motion*, the Law of the inspirational Heaven triad.

Her response to the guidance, "Carla, take this moment and expand on it," was to awaken to the second Law of the Human triad, *Chi Moves in the Space Between*. When she recognized that note as her "own pure creative potential," she opened up space inside of her psyche in which her chi could begin to flow once again.

She also recognized her creative potential was something "no one could take away" from her. With *that* realization, she began to rebuild the boundary that contained her "self," and so set the foundation for keeping her strength in the face of criticism. Reconnecting to her heart, Carla was able to define herself from the inside out. Part of this redefinition happened instantly, the rest has been an ongoing process over a number of years.

As Sharon Strand Ellison suggests in her book, *Taking the War Out of Our Words*, "Once we recognize our ability to work with our own energetic make-up, we realize we can refuse to take in any negative energy directed toward us."[1] For Carla, the blocks to the movement of chi within her, stemming from devastating criticism when she was a young adult, began to fall away. It became Carla's life practice "to hear what is authentic in the present moment as a pure note and expand on it."

The power to *Cultivate Discernment* is key to opening up the spaciousness within your psyche to allow for the movement of your life force and the expansion of your boundary, your wei chi.

Journal Entry: I have been thinking a lot lately about how often in my life I get stuck in low self-esteem. I think it's because I like the quality of "modesty" and don't quite know the difference. So what is the difference for me between modesty and low self-esteem? With modesty, my focus is not on myself; with low self-esteem, it is. When I genuinely feel humble, it is in the context of my awareness of my place in the larger scheme, in the web of life, my place as one cell in the great body of the universe. When I go into low self-esteem, I have no place in that larger context. I feel like I don't belong. This is important. I value my modesty as a Taoist virtue. I have continued to work to shift my low self-esteem to appropriate or rightful self-esteem while also celebrating my capacity to feel awe-filled humility within the vastness of creation.

Many people, from the time they were children, suffer from low self-esteem due to criticism and abuse from adults. Others enter young adulthood with excited anticipation, only to be beaten down then. I have a friend who won awards for her creative writing as a child and young adult but didn't write another word for 20 years after she was harshly criticized by two professors in graduate school. Yet, all of us, like Carla, have the ability to look for the pure note even in the midst of despair, and make our way back home.

Discernment in this context means cultivating your capacity to distinguish between what contributes to your growth and what doesn't, to recognize what feeds your energy as opposed to what drains it, to notice what keeps you in flow and what traps you in old patterns that no longer serve you. In other words, discernment helps you to transform your experience by hearing and attending to that note of authentic self that rings true.

I believe Carla's story is a vivid example of how the Human realm brings Heaven and Earth together. As Julia Cameron says, "Creativity is God's gift to us. Using our creativity is our gift back to God. …Our creative dreams and yearnings come from a divine source. As we move toward our dreams, we move toward our divinity."[2]

Paying Attention to the Impact of Our Choices

Hate cannot drive out hate; only love can do that. Hate multiplies hate, violence multiplies violence and toughness multiplies toughness, in a descending spiral of destruction. The chain reaction of evil must be broken, or we shall be plunged into the dark abyss of annihilation.
— *Dr. Martin Luther King, Jr.*

In order to be a conduit between Heaven and Earth, I believe you need to be able to establish which choices will best keep you aligned between your soul's purpose—the expression of Spirit as it comes to you—and your actions—the choices you make about what to do in your daily life. This is the underlying meaning and function of the practice, *Cultivate Discernment.* If we fail to practice discernment, we can easily be caught in reactive behavior, where each person in an interaction moves to the *lowest* common denominator.

I am fond of this well-known and oft-repeated story that seems relevant at this point.

What 'Wolf' Will You Feed?

One evening an old Cherokee told his grandson about a battle that goes on inside people. He said, "My son, the battle is between two 'wolves' inside us all. One is Evil. It is anger, envy, jealousy, sorrow, regret, greed, arrogance, self-pity, guilt, resentment, inferiority, lies, false pride, superiority, and ego. The other is Good. It is joy, peace, love, hope, serenity, humility, kindness, benevolence, empathy, generosity, truth, compassion and faith." The grandson thought for a minute and then asked his grandfather: "Which wolf wins?" The old grandfather simply replied, "The one you feed."

How many of us slide into resentment and anger that build over time, causing us to lose our integrity and openness? It can happen so slowly we don't even realize we have transformed ourselves into someone we don't recognize and do *not* want to be.

When you intentionally create a practice in which your day-to-day choices are based on healthy discernment, you establish the ground—prepare the Earth, so to speak—to clarify and live within your own boundaries, allowing chi to flow both within you and around you. In so doing, you bring Earth back to Heaven. Bringing Heaven to Earth and Earth to Heaven through the conduit of the Human realm creates a complete cycle that honors and enhances all aspects of our experience.

Invoking the Joy of the Human Realm

Once again, you can work with this Practice in four ways. The first is by "Embodying," which contains the physical exercises and Chi Kung forms that will create an energetic support system for the Human triad. Next, "Illuminating," includes meditations and chants based in the Human realm. The third category, "Accessing," contains witnessing exercises that ground the Human triad themes in daily life. Finally, "Deepening" explores how the discernment of your boundaries can support you as you open the internal space that will enhance your expression.

Warm-Ups/Stretches

The following stretches are specifically intended to open the lung meridian and release the heart chakra. They are especially useful if you've been feeling depressed, burdened, or at the mercy of your own brain mutter. When you are feeling shut down, your shoulders will tend to bow forward, as though "circling the wagons" to protect your heart. Opening the pectorals and relaxing the chest will give your body the opportunity and space to open the chi and allow your problem-solving mechanism begin to work, reconnecting you to your natural relaxed and open state.

Sand Angel

1. Lie on your right side. Bend your top (left) knee and place it on the floor in front of you. You may place a cushion under your head and/or your knee if this is more comfortable for your neck and back.

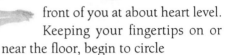

2. Extend your arms straight out in front of you at about heart level. Keeping your fingertips on or near the floor, begin to circle your top (left) arm up over your head. Follow your hand with your eyes. Allow your chest to open as you continue to circle your hand around behind you so that you are looking back over your shoulder with your back in a "cross stretch."

   Note: Depending on how flexible your back is, you may find that as your arm circles up or to the area behind you, your hand leaves the floor. Allow this to happen while keeping the arm heavy, so that you don't strain or over-twist your back or shoulder. Make sure your left shoulder is dropped as close to the floor as is comfortable or so you don't strain the top of your shoulder blade. Follow the limits of what feels comfortable and easeful in your body.

3. Continue to circle your arm, bringing your hand down to your hip. Do three circles in one direction, and then reverse the circle, bringing your hand down to your hip first, then circling up past your back, over your head, coming back around to the other hand.

4. Roll onto your left side and repeat circles in each direction with your right arm.

   Variation (for shoulder or back injury): If you are working with an injured shoulder or back, you can do this exercise by lying in position and raising your elbow with your hand hanging down. Gently move the elbow in small circles so the arm rotates slightly inside of the shoulder socket. Avoid pushing into any resistance and straining in your shoulder. The sensation should feel easeful.

Opening the Gates of Joy

1. Stand in a doorway with your feet slightly apart, facing out as though you were about to step through the door. Place your right hand on the doorjamb. Holding the doorjamb, take a step directly forward with your right foot until you feel a stretch across your pectoral muscles along the right side of your chest.

2. Once you step forward, make sure you relax your shoulder blades down your back so your right shoulder does not come forward or rise up and strain your neck. Keep your back vertical, and be careful not to twist your waist. If you feel a strain anywhere in your body, lighten up the stretch. It should feel like a pleasant pull across your chest.

3. Exhale while keeping your body aligned from the soles of your feet through the top of your head. Keep your knees soft, your lower back and buttocks relaxed, and imagine that your sitz bones are connected to your heels. Raise the crown of your head. Breathe deeply 1–3x.

Turn around and do the same thing with the left arm.

Embodying Joy of the Human Triad with Applied Chi Kung

The following exercises will help you to embody the information and energy intrinsic to the Human triad: the Law, *Chi Moves in the Space Between,* the Principle, *Boundaries Dissolve Barriers,* and the Practice, *Cultivate Discernment.* Notice which exercises most interest you. Although I have arranged them in a progressive order that I believe will make them accessible, feel free to choose your own order.

Stance Preparation—Aligning Heaven and Earth (Level I)

All of the following forms are done in a *Modified Horse Stance.* (p. 87) Here is a short warm-up to increase your ability to feel centered in your *Horse Stance.*

Centering for Horse Stance

1. Stand with your feet about hip distance apart, knees very slightly bent. Lift your toes off the floor for a moment, then spread them out and put them down on the ground again. Feel your weight distributed evenly

between your big toe, your little toe and your heel. The main require-
ment here is to find a stance that is balanced and relaxed.

2. Imagine the crown of your head lifting up to the sky above. At the same
time, picture your tailbone reaching like a long tail down to the earth.
Feel your feet firmly planted on the ground as though you were standing
in sand.

3. Slowly shift your weight from one foot to another. As you transfer your
weight from side to side, keep your spine vertical so you don't tilt or
bend at the waist. Keep the backs of your knees lightly relaxed so you
do not feel any strain in them. Shift from side to side about 9x or more.

4. Continuing to keep your spine aligned from the top of your head to
your tailbone, rock your weight forward and back so you balance first
on the balls of your feet, then on your heels. Again do not bend from the
waist. Rather, move your whole torso forward, then back. Repeat 9x or
more.

5. Continuing to maintain your alignment, move your weight in a circle,
shifting your weight first onto one foot, then to the balls of your feet,
then to the second foot and finally to your heels. Remember to keep
your spine vertical and your feet "planted in sand." Imagine that the top
of your head has a feather or paintbrush coming out of your crown and
that you are drawing a small circle in the air directly above you. Don't
go so far in your circle that you feel like you are losing your balance or
your heels or toes lift off the ground. Circle your weight 9x in one direction, then circle 9x in the opposite direction.

6. At the end of your 18 circles, bring your weight back to the center of
your feet, balanced again between the big toe, little toe and heel of each
foot. Feel the connection between your bubbling wells points (kidney
1's) and the earth below.

Chi Kung to Embody the Law *Chi Moves in the Space Between*

The following two forms work with developing your awareness of
chi as it moves through space within your body and its cells. *The Space
Shake* is a non-traditional way to generate a feeling of open space in your
body. *As Above, So Below* works to mindfully increase your awareness and
sensation of the power within that space.

The Space Shake: A "Spontaneous Chi Kung" Form

This first exercise contains an improvisational approach to moving chi. Adapted from a longer Kundalini practice, the *Space Shake* allows for a gentle release of tension in your muscles, aligning your skeleton as well as activating the flow of endorphins. You may enjoy this practice even more if you put on some lively music, or you may prefer to do it in silence.

The Form

1. Stand in *Modified Horse Stance*, keeping your feet planted and your spine aligned. Allow your body to begin to bounce up and down, in whatever ways or directions you feel moved to go. *Stay gentle with the movement.* You're not trying to shake out energy that is "bad." Rather, you are feeling for how the bones of your skeleton are balanced and for the sensation of the space within your joints. Imagine your bones are dancing, one on top of another. Shift your weight, let your tailbone wiggle and your head move around in whatever way it may move spontaneously. Allow your body to just relax, and enjoy a moderate movement. Let your arms swing and shake out your wrists and your tailbone guide your spine. As you play with this, your goal is not to try to "shake out" tension or force any structural change like "cracking" with your movement, although this might spontaneously happen. The only "rule" here is to stay centered on your feet. Every now and then, lift one heel or foot, then the other and shake them out, moving them around.

2. You may find that you can increase the sensation of opening space in your body if you also make some sighs, tones, or sounds of release. The Kundalini Yoga recommendation for this particular exercise is 15 minutes. If that feels too long, I recommend that you let your bones dance, your body shake for a minute or so, or the length of a song.

3. Stop moving, place your hands on your lower *tan tien*, and bring your focus back to your breath, feeling the sensation of chi as it moves within the space of your cells.

As Above, So Below

As Above, So Below is a traditional exercise common to several different styles or systems of Chi Kung. This form increases your ability to embody the Law *Chi Moves in the Space Between* as you begin to palpably sense the energy in the space both within and around your body.

The Form

1. Stand in a *Modified Horse Stance*. Soften your knees and relax your lower back so your tailbone hangs down toward the earth. Take a moment to breathe.

2. Rub your hands together briskly until the friction between your palms creates some warmth. Now cup your hands together, palms slightly apart, creating a hollow space between them. See if you notice a kind of warmth or a tingling sensation between your palms. If you don't feel any sensation at all or can't sustain the feeling between your hands, rub them together again until you do. Then cup your hands again.

3. Once you can feel some kind of sensation between your two cupped hands, slowly move them apart, keeping your palms turned toward one another. Sustain an awareness of that energy between your hands as they move further apart. If you don't continue to feel a connection, try bringing the hands a little closer together or rub your hands together again, generating more heat and then try it again. (When you are first practicing this exercise, it's more important to feel the energy between

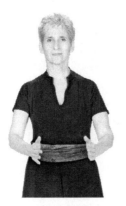 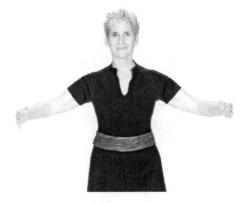

the two hands than it is to feel it continue as you move your hands outward.)

4. Move your hands in and out, toward and away from one another, palms in, as though you were playing an accordion. Notice if the quality of the sensation of energy shifts or changes as your palms get closer and further apart. Does it feel more intense and warmer as your hands come together? More stretched and cooler as they move apart? Or does it feel the same? There's no right answer or particular way you are "supposed to" experience the chi here. Just notice what you notice.

Chi Kung to Embody the Principle
Boundaries Dissolve Barriers

The two following Chi Kung forms generate waves of energy to establish healthy boundaries that both protect you and connect you with your environment. As these waves become stronger, you'll be increasingly able to expand to meet whatever challenges you may face.

Pebble in the Lake[3]

This form creates a ripple effect, which allows your energy to expand out around you in ever-widening concentric circles. Since we are energetic beings, it follows that we can both send and receive energy. As you work to increase your flow of chi with this form, your intention has a ripple effect, impacting those around you. When practicing this form, I have experienced, more often than "coincidence" would indicate, that, barking dogs have quieted down or neighborhood cats have appeared, lying down to soak up the chi bath. Also, students report that, when having a difficult interaction at work, if they do *Pebble in the Lake* either in their mind, or during a bathroom break, the energy of the interaction shifts. (Sometimes we joke about starting a "bathroom break" Chi Kung class.)

The Form

1. Stand in a *Modified Horse Stance*. Soften your knees and feel the connection between your sitz bones and your heels.

2. *Inhale* —

Physical: Draw your hands in toward one another in a parallel position in front of your lower *tan tien*.

Focus: As your hands come into position, imagine gathering and consolidating your energy in the belly.

3. *Exhale* —

Physical: Leading with the tips of your middle fingers and continuing to keep your palms turned down, move your hands straight ahead away from your body, belly level.

Focus: Imagine that you have dropped a pebble into the "lake" of your pelvis and energy begins to ripple out from your center.

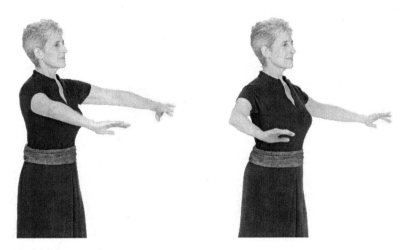

4. Exhale (continued)—

Physical: Leading with the outside edge of your wrists (pinky finger side), circle your hands away from one another and out to the sides as though you were gliding your palms over the surface of the ripples.

Focus: Picture ripples of energy spreading around you in wider and wider circles as a result of having dropped the pebble into the water. Let the ripples extend out in concentric circles as far as you want to imagine. They might extend just beyond your fingertips to the edges the room, the outskirts of your town, across country or ocean, even out to planets or galaxies beyond.

5. Inhale —

Draw your hands in toward one another in front of your lower *tan tien*, completing the circle. Then begin again.

I recommend doing at least 9 repetitions of *Pebble in the Lake*, breathing deeply as the ripples of chi expand around you. You may want to gradually extend the ripples during each repetition or keep them within the same parameters. When you finish, place one hand over the other on your lower abdomen (*tan tien*) and breathe.

Wei Chi[4]

As described in Chapter Four, *wei chi* is protective energy that is open, expansive and assertive—as opposed to defensive and shut down. *Wei chi* creates a potent emission that enhances the warm energy field around you, often referred to as an aura. Sometimes interpreted as "outer chi," this form blends yin and yang energy. It is the same warmth or tingling that you focused on feeling in your hands during *As Above, So Below*. With this practice, you permit that field of energy to radiate all around your body.

Before beginning, place your hands on your lower *tan tien* and breathe. Let your solar plexus soften and open. Take a moment to listen for and acknowledge what you know to be true about yourself. Imagine you are in your most open, trusting, and empowered place. This is the energy that you will focus on circulating around your body.

The Form

1. Stand in *Modified Horse Stance*. Bring your attention to the hollows or indents right below the center of the ball of each foot (kidney 1 point or "bubbling wells"). Picture these points connecting down into the ground. Imagine that your legs are like two straws drawing energy up from deep within the earth through each K1 point.

2. *Inhale* —

Cross your wrists one over the other (it does not matter which wrist is on top) at the level of your belly, palms turned in, elbows slightly bent. Imagine energy rising from the earth up your legs to your abdomen, then continuing to move up the centerline of your body. Allow your hands to be carried up by the ascending movement of chi coming up from below, as though they are riding a geyser, until they reach the crown of your head, the *Baihui* point. Then let the energy continue to rise straight above your head.

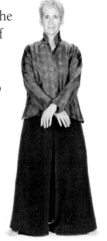

3. *Exhale* —

Circle your arms away from one another, stretching out to the sides, then slowing dropping them until they are down by your pelvis.

4. Crossing your wrists again, practice the circles 3x. (You can alternate which wrist is on top, if you like.) After your third circle, complete the sequence

by bringing your arms down by your sides and making fists with your hands. Place your thumbs on the inside of your fists. Stretch your fists straight down by your legs, imagining yourself grounding deep into the earth. (*Note:* This is a "Chi Kung" fist; please be aware this is *not* a fist you would make for a punch, as you would risk breaking your thumb. In this case, enclosing your thumb in your hand represents holding or containing your Spirit.)

5. Release your fists as you turn your waist to the left so your upper torso is rotated and you are looking to the left. Be careful not to twist either your knees or your pelvis. Using the same movement as before, cross your wrists towards the left of your lower abdomen and circle your arms up the center of your body and out to the sides. Now your circle will be diagonal to the first circle. Repeat 3x. Once again, make two fists with your thumbs on the inside and ground your energy, picturing your roots going deep into the earth.

6. Turn your waist so you're looking in the opposite direction, to the right. Repeat the sequence of circling your arms up and out on the second diagonal circle 3x. Finish by grounding with your fists again, sending your roots deep in the earth.

After you practice *Pebble in the Lake* and *Wei Chi*, stand still for a moment. Place your hands on your lower *tan tien*. Close your eyes and focus on your breath. Visualize, for a moment, the shapes you have made in the air around you with these last two forms. By doing horizontal circles of energy around your lower *tan tien* with *Pebble in the Lake* and then three vertical circles with *Wei Chi*—including one lateral and a left and a right diagonal circle—you have created a bubble of energy around your whole body. Doing these two Chi Kung exercises together creates an energy field that is identical to one of the designs sometimes used to represent an atom. Watch or feel yourself breathing here at the center of an expansive and powerful field of energy.

Chi Kung to Embody the Practice *Cultivate Discernment*

The Fountain

The *Fountain* increases your ability to be clear about your boundaries—your sense of self—and what diminishes or enhances your power. Particularly useful in the realm of communication, the *Fountain* is best used prior to an interaction with someone with whom you are experiencing conflict, when you'd like to be able to both listen and speak from a heart-centered, empowered place. (Of course, you would probably not actually do a Chi Kung form while in conversation—it would be distracting, to say the least, to wave your arms around while talking!). You can practice this form before entering any situation that makes you feel anxious. You can also picture yourself continuing to move your *Fountain* energy internally even during actual conversations. As is true with *Wei Chi*, the *Fountain* keeps you grounded by emanating a protective energy.

Dr. Khaleghl Quinn, from whom I learned the *Fountain*, describes this form in this way:

> The Fountain refers to four things:
>   a. an ability to bring that which is within out into the public domain;
>   b. the ability to recycle any given amount of energy; and, as a result of this recycling,
>   c. to tap an apparently endless supply of energy; rejuvenation, hence the fountain of youth;
>   d. to join forces with a different personality type, a different element, and to flow with the intent of that different point of view; then to return to one's own perspective enriched with more information.
>
> Successful communication is the purpose of the Fountain and results when we listen deeply to ourselves and to the hearts of others, sharing our energy with them. This energetic exchange also extends to places, animals and things. Whenever we are communicating, hearing the other person's intent and making known ours, we are exercising the Fountain.[5]

In difficult interactions with other people, you increase your ability to listen to what is behind their tone and words, regardless of how they are expressing themselves, and distill the content of what you are hearing down to its essence. Simultaneously you connect in a powerful way to your own truth and respond accordingly. This process transforms knee-jerk reactions in the face of adversity into heart-felt response.[6] In terms of intention, the *Fountain* does more than generate a process that distills information as it is coming to you. It creates an energetic netting or web that "separates the wheat from the chaff," so that you pay attention to what is useful, while allowing that which is not useful to be filtered out of your consciousness.

The Form

Stand in *Modified Horse Stance*.

Inhale —

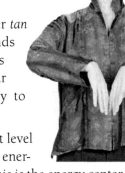

Physical: Start at the level of your lower *tan tien*, turning the backs of your hands towards one another, with the fingers pointing down, Draw the backs of your wrists up the centerline of your body to about chin level.

Focus: As you draw energy up to throat level from the lower *tan tien*, you are bringing energetic support up to the throat chakra. This is the energy center from which you speak your truth.

Exhale —

Physical: Leading with your little finger and letting your palms turn forward (outward), circle your hands away from one another and out to the sides, spreading your fingers apart. Keep your elbows bent and near your body and your fingers apart, as you circle your hands back down to your lower *tan tien*, returning to your starting place with the backs of the hands turned towards each other, fingers pointing down. As you circle your arms, keep the fronts of your shoulders relaxed, as though your clavicles are smiling. (Note: Similar to the technique of *Wei Chi,* you will once again be circling your hands and arms by coming up the centerline of your body and out to the sides. However, in the *Fountain*, the circles that you are making are a little smaller and closer to the body, extending outward from the elbows, rather than from the shoulder, with a full-length extension of your arms.)

Focus: In Dr. Quinn's teaching, each finger corresponds to the different elements of earth, water, fire, air, and ether, creating an energetic protective filter, which allows in information or energy that helps you grow and filters out whatever drains you or keeps you stuck. As your hands circle out to the sides, you are opening the space by your ears, as though you were describing really big "Dumbo" (elephant) ears, increasing your ability to hear the intention behind someone's words or tone. As your hands come back together, imagine that you are consolidating your own thoughts and summoning the energy to speak from your center.

Repeat 9x or more.

Steep the Tea

As you did in the previous Practice, *Embrace Wholeness,* (p. 94), take a moment to lie down to rest and "steep the tea." This grounds the energy you have generated with your Chi Kung practice. When you lie down on your back for a few moments and then turn onto your side and curl up, you are allowing your body to simulate sleep. Studies have shown we best absorb learning something new or taking something in when we sleep. When you *Steep the Tea*, you are essentially giving your body the message to absorb the information, "fooling" it into thinking this, like sleep time, is the time of great integration.

Tapping

After *Steeping Tea,* complete your Chi Kung practice with the *Tapping/Patting* exercise described on page 95 of Chapter 5 to "seal in" the energy you have moved.

Illuminating the Human Triad: Meditation

This section includes meditations and chants based in the Human triad. To begin, I would like to offer some other options for grounding and centering your body right before you meditate.

Body Centering for Meditation (Sitting)

1. Feel your sitz bones connected to the ground or chair on which you are sitting.
2. Slowly rock forward and back on your sitz bones. Return to your center of balance. Breathe.
3. Shift your weight from side to side, from one sitz bone to the other. Return once more to center. Breathe.
4. Circle your weight from one point to the next, by shifting onto one sitz bone, then back to the tailbone. Move to the other sitz bone, then forward over your perineum. You are circling the perimeter of your base, your foundation. As you circle, feel the crown of the head lifted up towards the sky, opening like a sunflower to the sun. Do this 3x. Breathe.
5. Circle in the opposite direction 3x. Come back to center. Breathe.

Body Centering for Meditation (Lying Down)

If you cannot sit comfortably for a length of time, try this grounding and centering preparation for lying on your back.

1. Lie on your back. Bend your knees and place your feet on the ground next to your buttocks. Let your bones drop down towards the ground and imagine an opening of space between each bone and joint.

2. As you lie there, wiggle your tailbone a little, letting that releasing motion travel up your spine. Gently rock your head from side to side as though you were saying "no." Keep your movement small within the area of contact where your head is touching the floor.

3. Next nod up and down as though you were saying "yes," again keeping the movement small and comfortable.

4. Last, circle around the perimeter of that point of contact, where the back of your head meets the surface your head. Circle 3x in one direction, then 3x in the other.

5. Do the same thing now with your hips. Begin by gently rocking your pelvis from one hip to the other, from side to side. As you did with your head, keep the movement contained within the point of contact where the back of your pelvis is touching the floor.

6. Rock your pelvis up and down, going from the small of your back to the tailbone. Do not push or force a stretch here, but, instead, explore your range of motion within this contained area.

7. Circle the circumference of the point of contact where the back of your pelvis is touching the floor, moving your weight from your left hip to your tailbone, over to the right hip and back to the small of your back. Circle 3x in one direction, and then reverse directions for another 3 circles.

Quantum Meditation

This meditation works with the theme of the Law, *Chi Moves in the Space Between*. Take your time as you travel in your mind's eye into your core essence.

Note: As I described in Chapter 5, you may read this yourself, and then meditate with whatever images you remember, or have a friend read it to you as you meditate, or record it and play it back. Lightly place the tip of your tongue on the roof of your mouth behind your front teeth.

Spend a moment keeping your focus on your breath as it moves in and out of your body. Notice the cool air as you inhale, then exhale the warmed air that has circulated through your lungs. As you breathe, be aware that your body is made up of cells, microcosmic entities of space and particles. These cells that are your body are made of more than 99% space. Within that space live particles. Each particle is subsequently made up of space and more particles. In turn, each of those particles is essentially space.

Breathe into the space that is your body and imagine your life force, chi moving freely, bringing you vitality and connection. As you inhale, breathe in the molecules of oxygen exhaled by the plants in the environment around you. As you breathe out, return molecular energy to those plants in the form of carbon dioxide.

Breathe into the cells that compose every hair on your body, then to the cells that are your skin. Through your imagination, enter deeper into the spaciousness of your cells. Travel into the lining of your veins and the blood that moves within them. Picture the spacious cells of your lymph system, your muscles, your organs. Breathe into the cellular space of your skeleton, the bones of your body. Move your consciousness even deeper into the cellular space that is at the very marrow of your bones.

You are pure energy, particles moving and interacting within a vast microcosm of space. Breathe. As you continue to move deeper down into the quantum field, feel your physical being made up of space and particles perceivable through their relationship to one another. In movement, they encase clouds of possibility.

Picture that you have traveled down to your very core, the essence of the cosmic intelligence that holds us together in this particular shape at this particular moment in time—the mystery. Breathe into that source. Listen for the bountiful unending essence that permeates you from the quantum field, through the subatomic structure into your cells, into the marrow of your bones all the way through your body, out to the hair on your skin. Picture that energy radiating within you, above and below you, all around you. You may see this energy as light, warmth, sound, vibration, movement, or some combination. Allow your awareness of chi to fill you, empower you, remind you that you are, in your essence, made of the same material as the entire cosmos that surrounds and permeates our planet. Breathe. Through the very matter of your being and through the aliveness of your Spirit, you are interconnected with the vast mystery that is Consciousness.

Solar Plexus Bowl

This meditation is especially useful when your body tightens up because you feel like you need to protect yourself. The concept that your boundaries and your protection come from openness and expansive space requires a paradigm shift that your body needs to embrace as much as your mind. The following sitting meditation practice comes from the work of the integrative healer/teacher Damaris Jarboux, co-founder with James MacRitchie of the Body-Energy Center and director of The Center Place, both in Boulder, Colorado.

In her work, Jarboux has explored the impact and vital importance of relaxing and opening the solar plexus. She describes the solar plexus as the portal that emits protective energy, which she poetically describes as an egg of light. This "egg" has a permeable shell that acts as a filter to keep out what you don't need and bring in what you do need. In other words, this protective energy is the same as I experienced when I was walking down the street and a man tried to grab my breast—it is the field of *wei chi*.

Akin to the third chakra, the solar plexus is sometimes referred to as the body-soul connection. In a workshop, Jarboux compared the reaction of a stressed solar plexus to the eye of a camera closing its shutter. When the solar plexus becomes tight and stuck, it cuts off the flow of wei chi, the outer energy that is the source of *actual* protection. On the other hand, with the practice of the *Solar Plexus Bowl* meditation, as your solar plexus becomes relaxed and open, you transform stagnant chi so that it radiates through your wei chi as the whole and integrated self contained by your boundaries.

I think you'll find this meditation practice works extremely well in conjunction with the practice of *Wei Chi*. In fact, I frequently sit with this meditation before practicing the standing form.

Dr. Jarboux has generously given me permission to quote from her handout, *The Solar Plexus Bowl Practice*. What follows are her verbatim directions for this powerful practice.

The Practice
by Damaris Jarboux

This practice can be done in any position, but it is a good practice to do in bed before going to sleep at night or getting up in the morning. It takes 10 minutes at first.

- Resting your mind in center, become aware of your solar plexus— as if you were witnessing from the center

- As you exhale, imagine you are sending your breath there.

- Feel the area; notice the quality, sensation or image that is there.

- Lightly place your hands on your solar plexus with your fingertips in a straight line from your navel to the xyphoid (at the bottom of your breast bone), right hand on top.

- Your thumbs are not used except as a vent. Your fingertips are just lightly touching your body (wearing clothes is fine).

- Imagine a bowl inside your solar plexus area facing up; the surface of your skin is the top of the bowl

- Let the energy of your fingertips sink down into the area like they were sinking into the bottom of the bowl

- Watch (from your place of rest in center) and feel your **willingness** to allow this area of your body to soften, relax and begin to open like the eye of a camera. Tell your willingness to let go of the habit of over-protecting and unnecessary guarding and shielding. You are filtering your own light out by doing that. Effort/work (pushing your fingers way in) won't help, it will only close tighter.

- You will start to feel a **physical response** as your body begins to let go of your unconscious stress response and sink slowly into relaxation response.

- Keeping your hands in place, imagine (see it or just think it) an egg of light at the edge of your personal field, at least three feet out. It is a permeable shell that filters out what you don't need and brings in what you do need. (This is not about your personal wants and desires, but about your soul's needs). See and feel it behind you, in front, to the sides, above and below you. Like a large egg of white/golden light white light surrounding and protecting your body and your personal energy cocoon, this field is real, and it gets stronger every time you think about it.

- Now, remembering the egg of light that is your **real filter**, proceed with willingness to break up the **false filter** that you're holding in your solar plexus. Move your hands so that your fingertips rest on either side at the base of your rib cage. Again, let the energy from your fingertips sink in like your fingers were growing longer and sliding down the sides of the bowl to the bottom, meeting in the middle. They are "breaking up" the filter pattern/habit in that part of the bowl nearest your chest.

- Move your hands so your fingertips are on each side, directly below your nipples and below your ribcage. Again, let your "energy fingers" sink down the sides of the bowl, breaking up the filter/pattern at the part of the bowl to your sides. Let yourself really feel and image this happening. [**Note from Vicki:** I have had some students who prefer to visualize those old patterns softening and releasing, rather than "breaking up." Use whatever image is the easiest for you to allow the shift of releasing the blockage to happen.]

• Move your hands around the bowl so your index fingers meet in your navel and your fingertips fan out on either side of your navel. Again, let your fingers grow and sink down the sides of the bowl to the bottom, breaking up the pattern of over-protection at the area of the bowl closest to your navel. There is no one way to do this, just "walk" your hands (separately or together) around the bowl, breaking up the pattern. Stay in willingness, not effort.

• Come back to the mid-line (first position) again with fingertips in a straight line, navel to xyphoid. Sink in again.

When you're ready, take a deep breath in and as you exhale, let your mind lead your breath down and out your solar plexus. Keep doing this as you draw your hands off your body—drawing this old pattern of energy out. Be glad to let it go. Each time you exhale, fill your solar plexus with breath and light, and keep drawing your hands from your solar plexus bowl out. You can even circle your hands out clockwise.

There is nothing "bad" leaving during this practice, just an old habit of protection that has been subconsciously keeping your body in stress response and weakening your constitution to some degree, because it was filtering your own light from **full** descent into your physical body. This is not just the cauldron/chakra that we are engaged with, it is a much bigger center, the only "eye" of its kind in your body. Some version of this eye and egg practice was part of the esoteric tradition of every indigenous culture that survived; we have forgotten its importance. Remember, once you have developed this process, it is faster and you can do it with your mind. In Chi Kung, we understand that the mind can lead the chi and also the chi can lead the mind. If something happens to you that is a shock or trauma, this eye will probably close—it is supposed to. But it will open as soon as things settle; if you're doing the practice, it won't remain stuck closed.

If you do this daily (for 10 minutes) or two times daily, it will entrain your energy-body to respond quicker and deeper each time. The egg (the real filter) will get stronger and your constitution (elements, organs, meridians) will strengthen. Gradually, your "Solar Plexus Eye" will be more and more open until it functions at 80-100% all the time instead of 0-30% like most people. Your whole life will feel and be different! I guarantee it—if you **do** it, because I have developed this practice for 15 years with people both in treatment and teaching them to do it themselves—I can **always** tell when someone is doing the practice. It is reflected in body, emotions, thoughts, work, relationships—their whole life.

When you have fully embodied this and see it in your life—teach it to someone else. If you know a receptive teenager, pass it along. It will be an invaluable tool for life![7]

A Standing Practice for the Solar Plexus Bowl

As I worked with Jarboux's *Solar Plexus Bowl*, I decided to create a standing Chi Kung application, bringing together *Aligning Heaven and Earth* (Level 1)[8] with the *Solar Plexus Bowl* meditation. The focus of this practice is to remember to keep your solar plexus open and relaxed, radiating wei chi even when you have been pushed off-center or feel out of balance. I put it here because there are many instances in the course of a day that can increase our stress levels, throw us off-center and make our bodies tight. Reactions to everyday occurrences that we may think of as mundane, such as an erratic driver's road rage, a child whining for attention at just the wrong moment, unwelcome news from a co-worker, even a depressing newspaper headline—may be easily forgotten by your conscious mind but still cause your body to react, your solar plexus to tighten and your wei chi to diminish. This standing form gives you a practice to remember you can restore your chi in almost any environment.

Aligning Heaven and Earth: Level 2

1. Standing in *Modified Horse Stance*, place your fingertips lightly on your solar plexus. Relax and breathe. Allow your solar plexus to become very soft in the same way you did with the *Solar Plexus Bowl* practice. Do not press your fingers so far into your solar plexus that you feel yourself begin to tighten and resist. Rather, imagine that your solar plexus is relaxed and glowing.

2. Repeat the same sequence that you did in the previous exercise, *Aligning Heaven and Earth* (Level 1). Shift your weight first from side to side, then forward and back, finishing with a circle 9x in each direction. This time, however, take yourself to the outside edge of your balance. Pay attention to when your solar plexus begins to tighten or push against your fingers. When it does, slow down and come back from the edge of your balance until you can feel your solar plexus soften again. See how far off balance,

right to the edge of your comfort zone, you can go *while still maintaining a relaxed solar plexus*. It's more important for your solar plexus to stay open and relaxed than it is to test how far off center you can go. The purpose is to train your body to stay open and relaxed, allowing your chi to continue to flow through space, even when you do feel off-balance.

Three Realm Toning: Level 2

As with the first level of *Three Realm Toning* in the *Embrace Wholeness* chapter (p. 100), this practice uses the vibration of sound to stimulate the energy in each *tan tien*: Shen (Heaven realm), Tai (Human realm) and Jing (Earth realm).

This series is best done as a standing/walking meditation, although you are welcome to adjust it for any physical limitations you may have.

Note: As you did in the first level of this meditation, relax your throat, allowing your breath to be supported by your belly as you make the sound. If your throat starts to feel tight or to hurt, reduce your volume. Sound these tones at whatever pitch, length and number of times is comfortable for you.

1. Stand in a *Modified Horse Stance*. Begin with the lower *tan tien*, *Jing*—the Earth realm in your body. As though you were embracing the trunk of a tree, circle your arms in front of you at a level between your belly and solar plexus. Point the tips of the fingers towards one another, without actually allowing them to touch. Keep your hands relaxed and your shoulders down and back. Visualize that your sitz bones are connecting to your heels, and that you have roots extending from your tailbone and your bubbling well points (the hollows below the center of the ball of each foot) down into the earth.
   a. Using the lower, deeper range of your voice, tone the syllable *om*. Feel the vibration of the sound traveling into the bones of your pelvis, legs and feet until you feel like you are shaking any stagnation loose. Repeat your tone 3–9x.
   b. After you have completed the sound, place your hands on your lower *tan tien* and breathe. Listen for a sensation of warmth or tingling in your lower body.
2. Shake out your arms and legs and walk around for a moment, feeling the contact of your feet with the ground.
3. Move your attention to your middle *tan tien*, *Tai*, the Human realm of your body. Stretch your arms straight out to the sides, anywhere between hip and shoulder height. How high you raise your arms isn't as important as keeping your neck and shoulders relaxed. Bring your arms

slightly forward in front so you can see them easily in your peripheral vision. If you begin to feel tense during the course of the sounding, lower your arms until they are at a level that feels comfortable. Gradually, over time, your stamina will build and you will be able to hold them higher.

    a. Using the middle range of your voice, tone the syllable *haaah* into your chest and upper back. Let the sound to vibrate the heart center of your body, and move down your arms out to the tips of your middle fingers. Repeat 3-9x.

    b. After you have completed the sound, place your hands on your heart chakra and breathe. Listen for a sense of tingling or vibration indicating the arrival of chi.

4. Shake out your arms and legs and walk around for a moment, keeping your attention on the center of your chest. Imagine your heart opening and connecting to the environment around you.

5. Move your attention to your upper *tan tien, Shen,* the Heaven realm in your body. Stretch your arms up over your head in a "V" shape, as though you were creating a large cup or chalice with your head in the middle of it.

    a. Using the high range of your voice, or *falsetto,* tone the syllable, "*sseeeeee,*" directing the sound to vibrate the bones of your head. Then let the sound travel up your arms and vibrate between your hands. Be sure to keep your jaw and the space between the eyebrows relaxed and open.

    b. After you have completed the sound, place your hands on the top of your head, or, if your arms are too fatigued, place your hands back on your lower *tan tien.* Keep your attention on the crown of your head and once again listen for a sensation of tingling or vibration in the bones of your skull. See if you can also perceive energy moving above your head.

6. Again, shake out your arms and legs and walk around, sensing the crown of your head and its connection to the sky.

You may complete this chanting meditation by doing the "*Tapping*" (*patting*) exercise described on page 95.

Journal

Jot down any insights, images, impressions or thoughts you experienced as you chanted.

Accessing the Human Triad: Choosing Joy in Your Daily Life

The following exercises are designed to cultivate your discernment during times when your life force feels blocked. What choices might you make to open space, move chi, and reestablish your boundaries? You may want to begin by trying one of the following exercises for 5 minutes during the week ahead. As you enhance your mindfulness about your habits and reactions, you will have longer intervals of awareness without having to sacrifice time to do the other things you need to do in a day. I highly recommend that you make a little time at the end of each day to note your observations in your journal.

Accessing the Space Between

As you move through your day, pause every once in a while to notice where your thoughts are going when you are between different tasks. Are you thinking about what you just did, what you are going to do next? Are you fretting about what you have yet to accomplish? Notice if you're feeling as though you are cramped in your thoughts and feelings or if your energy feels like it is flowing freely. If you're flowing freely, breathe into that awareness and enjoy! If you feel stressed, out of breath, or like there just isn't enough time, interrupt this momentum to take a few deep breaths to open to your inner place of stillness and allow chi to flow again in the "space between."

Accessing the Witness—Choosing Focus: Embracing or Resisting?

During the course of your day, take stock of a time when you feel, for example, interrupted or distracted by someone while you are trying to focus on something else. Once that distraction is over, take a moment to breathe into the stillness of the "space between," the present moment, the home of the Observer. As you breathe, relax your mind. Focus simply on your breath moving in and out. Notice, as if from outside of yourself, whatever you notice about how you are, your state of being after that interruption.

During this process, keep focusing on your breath. Breathe. Now ask yourself more specifically about what you're feeling and thinking. First, see if you are able to *not* be attached to your emotion or thoughts. Try not to analyze, justify, or push away the experience. Allow it. Witness from the Observer space: Are you embracing "what is" or resisting it? Are you still frustrated or distracted because of the interruption? Irritated with whoever interrupted you? You can ask yourself:

"Are my reactions a sign that I need to create clearer boundaries with this person?"

"Do I think it was a necessary interruption, yet still feel angry?"

"Do I believe I need to leave what I was doing to follow up with the person? If so, is that what I actually want to do, or not? If I do, is it a way to avoid my own task or is it where I 'need to be' right now?" Breathe.

"Is how I am feeling contributing to making a transition to what I need to be doing, or is it holding me back, keeping me distracted?"

"Do I want to keep thinking about what happened or am I ready to shift back to my original activity?"

"Is there another kind of response I'd like to cultivate in this situation? For future situations?"

It is vital to avoid judging yourself or thinking about what you "should" do. Rather, in order to cultivate discernment, merely practice making a choice based on your observations and/or desires now.

This exercise can help you draw upon the Heaven realm inside of you, as *Chi Moves in the Space Between,* to discern whether your chi is flowing or feels stagnant. This is a key to understanding and honoring your own boundaries, which is, in turn, a key to your health. Staying stuck in stagnant chi will not only prevent you from getting back on task after an interruption, it'll also stunt your emotional, intellectual, and even spiritual growth. Our lives are made up of how we handle each interaction, one by one.

How you respond to even a simple interruption can, over time, become a foundation for creating boundaries, not only with some other person—but also with yourself in regard to how you choose to use your own energy when life interrupts you. When you make the choice to set clear boundaries on your own use of energy so that you become responsive rather than reactive, you become able to embrace "what is" and move past it without getting stuck. When you do so, you allow chi to flow both within you and around you.

Accessing Joy

Imagine you have in your essence a wellspring of joy you can access at any moment. Even if you can't quite believe it because of difficulties or stresses you are experiencing, pretend that you do. Write the following question on a piece of paper and tape it next to your bed or on your bathroom mirror so you see it when you begin your day. "How will I access joy during my day today?" Make a point of reading it every morning when you wake up, and allow the inquiry to float in the back of your mind throughout the day. Before you go to sleep at night, reflect on when and how you succeeded on accessing your joy that day.

Accessing Grounding

Wake Up: When you wake up in the morning, place your hands in the middle of your chest over your thymus gland and your heart chakra. Circle your hands on your chest several times in each direction. Ask yourself, "What can I truly say I am grateful for today?" As each thought image or sound comes to you, take the time and space to breathe it in. Feel it.

Walking Tall: You may want to try out this exercise immediately and get up from wherever you may be reading. However, I recommend that after you've experienced it, you make a mental note to try it out during the week ahead.

During the course of your day, while you are doing some routine task like walking to your car or bus stop, standing in line, or washing the dishes, take about 5 minutes to divide your attention into two parts. Keep half of your attention on your task—whatever you need to pay attention to—and the other half on the alignment of your body as you do whatever you are doing. Where are you carrying your weight? Are you tilted forward on your feet or bottom? Are you resting back on your heels or tailbone?

Now picture yourself suspended between Heaven and Earth. Imagine that the roof of your mouth is lifted high like the ceiling in a cathedral and that your tailbone and sitz bones are grounded down into the earth. Feel gravity ground you through your feet at the same time that your crown opens to the heavens as a sunflower opens towards the sun.

Relax your jaw and the space between your eyebrows. As you continue your task, notice what happens to your lungs, to your ability to breathe as you sustain the image of being lifted up to the heavens and grounded by earth. What do you notice in your shoulders, your belly or any other areas of your body where you usually carry tension? As you inhale, expand your lungs all the way from your chest down to your belly, feeling the movement of your ribs. As you exhale, imagine the bones of your skeleton dangling easily from your skull and neck. Notice, as you breathe, whether or not you are pushing your ribs forward. If you are, bring them back into alignment and picture them hanging down from your shoulder blades.

Picture the top of your head as the bud of a flower opening to the sunlight at the same time you feel your feet, your "roots," sinking into the ground. Now notice what is happening inside your solar plexus. See if you can imagine that your solar plexus is relaxing and opening, supporting the center of your chest as your heart softens. Imagine that your heart is being fed and nurtured from the earth below. See if you can sustain this body awareness, your attention half out, half in for at least 5 minutes and play with increasing the amount of time you can hold it as you practice during the days ahead.

Deepening the Discernment of the Human Triad: Journal Exercises

Although I have suggested times for each of these rapid writes, as I did in the previous Practice chapter, feel free to write longer. You can use your discernment to decide! Again, the goal here is to strike a balance that allows you to listen more deeply to your guidance, yet not be so extensive or complex that you end up sabotaging yourself and not doing the exercise because you don't have time or feel overwhelmed. Do try to make your journaling be as effortless and as pleasurable as possible.

Invoking "Inter-being"

Recommended Time: 3 minutes

I feel most connected to myself, to others and to the world around me when I...

Easy Going

Recommended Time: 3 minutes

I feel most Alive and at ease with myself when I...

In My Wei Chi

Recommended Time: 3 minutes

If I had all of the time/space and resources that I needed, the gift I think I could offer to those around me is...

Discovering the Means

Recommended Time: 2 minutes each part

1. *One of my favorite ways to express myself is...*
2. *If I felt totally free to express myself fully, one thing I'd like to say is.... Another is...*

What Feeds Me? What Drains Me?

This journal exercise works specifically to cultivate discernment about your own choices.

Take a moment at the end of your day to sit quietly in a chair.

Breathe. Relax. Notice whether your mind is at peace or whether there are urgent matters calling for your attention—that phone call that must be made, the bill you forgot to pay, the chore that remains undone. Ask yourself if these are things you can put aside for a half-hour. If the answer is "absolutely not," come back to this exercise when the time is right. If the answer is "yes," then make an agreement with yourself that you'll attend to those other matters at another time. If you need to jot down a reminder to yourself to do so in your journal, do it now, then put it aside.

Now turn your attention to your body. Notice if your body feels aligned or slumped. Do you have energy, or do you feel depleted? Are you buzzing with thoughts that are inspiring? Do you feel stressed? Tired? Are you fatigued, yet relaxed? Content? Or are you exhausted? Just take a moment to take stock. Notice whatever you notice, feel whatever you feel. Do not try to change or fix anything—just notice where you are.

Bring your attention to the top of your head and the roof of your mouth. Imagine the crown of your head is lifting up towards the sun. Cast your thoughts back over the past few days or week. What's been going on? Notice what you feel, especially in your body, as different images and impressions move through you. Do your eyebrows or forehead contract? Are there moments when you tighten your jaw or clench your teeth? Do your shoulders begin to ache? Do you feel tension in the pit of your belly? Is your solar plexus tight or relaxed? Is your chest soft or constricted?

Are there images that pass through that bring a smile to your face or a sigh of release? Is there any moment where you feel a bubble of excitement at your core? Do not try to judge, talk yourself out of what you are feeling, or change anything for the moment. Simply notice it.

Be aware of what images or scenarios bring tension into your body—someone in your life who did or said something that made you feel discounted or diminished, a boss who was unreasonably demanding, a spouse who was insensitive or critical, a child who irritated you, pressure to meet a deadline, worries about What Might Happen.

Also be aware of images that bring feelings of peace or love into your body—a smile in response to something you did or said, the sound of a child's giggle of delight, a feeling of accomplishment, or a moment with your pet that made you laugh.

After you've completed your inner scan, open your eyes and your journal. First jot down all of the images that delighted you, brought a smile to your face or heart. Notice the qualities of these images: feelings of merriment, release, love, gratitude. Notice what you feel in your body as you bring focus to these images. Take a moment to appreciate yourself and these occasions.

Then take a fresh page and draw a line down the center of it. On the left side of the page, write down all of the images and thoughts that made you feel tight or tired, irritated, or depressed. Any images that interrupt your sense of well-being. Take your time and be thorough. Uncomfortable or even painful as these memories might be, see if you can welcome them as signposts to direct you back to your joy—even if it seems impossible at the moment. Let yourself become curious. Don't forget to breathe as you do this part of the exercise.

When you have completed the list, go to the right column. In this column, write the words "So what *do* I want?" On the other side of the line, go down the list you have written point by point. With this exercise, do not try to find solutions to the problems that brought you to this place. Rather, notice how the list on the left makes you feel and write down what you would prefer to feel.[9] For example:

What am I experiencing that I don't want?	*What do I want instead?*
I am so angry at Arnold for leaving such a mess in the kitchen	I want to experience reciprocity in all of my relationships
I feel uninspired and depressed at work	I want to find occasions in my life that inspire and excite me
I am uncomfortable in my body and feel unattractive	I want to feel my own vitality, to enjoy being in my body
I feel furious that my car broke down again!	I want to experience flow in my life, no matter what is going on

Once you have completed your lists, re-read the column on the right and, for the next few days, mull over how you want to feel, what you want to experience in those challenging situations. When you find your mind muttering about whatever may be making you feel bad or drained, see if you can recognize how these things might be signposts directing you to what you need to do. Notice what occurs in your life that fits what you *do* want. Jot those down in your journal at the end of the day. For example, "Arnold noticed that I had cleaned the kitchen and thanked me for the first time ever!" Or "I just met this fabulous woman who is going to teach me how to..." Or "Today, I chose to climb the stairs instead of take the elevator. I felt my muscles working and am going to try to do it more often." These observations will help you recognize change and progress toward your desired goals.

Conclusion: Making Choices with Intention

Cultivate Discernment is a practice of intention, of learning to distinguish between what feeds your joy and what blocks it. This isn't always only a matter of what you prefer or what "makes you happy." Rather, this Human triad Practice teaches you to notice what allows your chi to flow and what does not. As you increase your ability to discern, you'll be on a path that gives you the spaciousness for individuation, self-definition.

On a physical plane, pay attention to your solar plexus as the key to enhancing the robustness of your wei chi. Ask yourself from time to time whether your solar plexus is tight, preventing you from emanating your power. Notice other body signals that tell you whether you are accepting or resisting "what is." Have you been gritting your teeth during the day? Feeling extra tension in your shoulders or back? On the emotional plane, see if you are carrying burdens of over-responsibility and resentment on your shoulders or where you feel stuck in your life.

On the mental level, listen to your brain mutter. If you are looping over some problem again and again, take a moment to breathe, open space in your mind so you can access your problem-solving mechanism more easily. Finally, on the spiritual plane, imagine yourself as one cell within infinite consciousness, a specific facet on the Cosmic Gem. What gifts do you bring to the world around you? Being a Parent? An Artist? Some form of service? The list is infinite.

Through this process of discernment you most effectively act as a conduit between Heaven and Earth, between guidance/inspiration and what you manifest, because you will make choices that come from your heart. The heart is not only the central chakra of the seven-chakra system, it is the most radiant of all the energy centers, the place where Heaven and Earth conjoin.

When you intentionally align with your heart to inform and direct the choices you make every day, you will find a quality of spaciousness both in your inner life and in relationship to other people. Within that space, chi flourishes, bringing physical vitality and emotional equanimity. Hence you embody the Human triad Law *Chi Moves in the Space Between*.

Living in a mind- and heart-set where chi is moving through space, your boundaries become clear and effortless, creating new levels of connection within yourself and with the world around you. In this way, you embody the Human triad Principle *Boundaries Dissolve Barriers*.

In the Heaven triad, the lesson of the Practice, *Embrace Wholeness,* was to cultivate your Observer Self in order to balance polarities and so be able to live wholly in the experience of all-that-is. In the Human triad, the lesson of the Practice, *Cultivate Discernment,* is to make choices oriented in your heart. In so doing, you will find yourself consistently in alignment between guidance and manifestation, emanating Love, and walking a path that is an expansive expression of your life purpose.

PART III
The Body of Joy
Manifestation

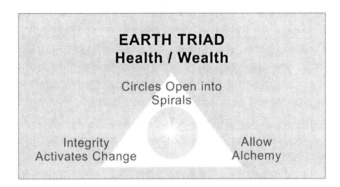

God bless the roots! Body and soul are one.
— *Theodore Roethke*

The Earth triad of the *Way of Joy* contains the Law, Principle, and Practice that ground the other two triads. On the Earth plane the inspiration from the Heaven triad and the application of the Human triad come to manifestation and we are called upon to "walk the talk." As Harriet Beinfeld and Efrem Korngold say in their book, *Between Heaven and Earth: A Guide to Chinese Medicine*, "I am the composer and the composed...the instrument and the player"[1] or, I am the *inspirer of* and the actual *creation from* that impulse. Here is where things we have envisioned become tangible. The Earth realm is where you co-create your life with Source.

At a primal level, the Earth realm includes the physical entity of our bodies, from the marrow in our bones to the hair on our skin. Our bodies come from the earth and return to her—we are the earth. Located in the pelvis, legs, feet, and extending three feet into the ground, the Earth realm emanates the qualities of wealth, health and power. It's also in the Earth realm that, as Dr. Quinn says, we have "a leg to stand on," where we "stand our ground" and back up our convictions. The Earth is also the source of nourishment, of the food that literally springs from it.

The Earth realm is not just a place where we manifest Heaven-inspired visions. Since the Earth realm includes an area that is three feet underground, it also encompasses what is happening "beneath the surface" or in the unconscious. Whereas the Heaven realm is the home to the intuitive "aha!," it's in the Earth realm that we access our instinct, that "gut feeling" that prompts us to make certain instant choices. Perhaps, for example, you cross the street when you sense some kind of energy you don't like in a person walking toward you or you spontaneously go to a show and unexpectedly run into just the person you need to see right now.

At the same time, the Earth realm gives us access to insights that have been buried deep in the psyche, that come to us in our sleep through our dreams. Unlike the visionary clarity and imaginative guidance that characterize information from the Heaven realm, our deepest fears and unremembered influences reside in the Earth realm.

The Earth realm includes all that has happened in the past, the influences and experiences of our childhood. This realm also includes our ancestry, our roots—both biological and spiritual—the genetic and cultural knowledge we inherit from our predecessors. When we summon the intention and the courage to bring past influences (both conscious and unconscious) to the surface, we are willing to encounter shame and discomfort and bring them to the light of awareness. Doing so creates the foundation for transformative healing. Examining roots and all that is attached to them is as essential as inspiration is in striving to achieve our dreams.

Heaven Aspect of the Earth Triad: *Circles Open Into Spirals*

As the Heaven aspect of the Earth triad, the Law, *Circles Open to Become Spirals,* provides the universal consciousness and guidance for this realm. It provides information we need to access and examine what has been buried. It is the guidance that moves us beyond the fear of opening Pandora's Box so that we can experience a deep examination of our own psyche as an exploration into freedom. In the process we can shift from shame and blame to strength and openness.

The Natural World is the inspiration this triad's Heaven aspect brings. Nature, of which humans are an element, is an unending cycle of life, death, and rebirth. Whether you believe in reincarnation or not, on a purely physical plane our actual bodies are born, live, then die and return to the earth as compost, which is in itself the source for new life. We cannot receive inspiration from the universe without honoring Nature's cycles.

Because we live in a cyclical environment, we inevitably discover patterns of repetition as our lives unfold. Circles of experience and response loop around again and again with essentially the same refrain—"Here we go again." On a biological level, these experiences cause the neurons of the brain to wire together to make associative connections that color our perceptions and choices. As Joe Dispenza says in his book, *Evolve Your Brain: The Science of Changing Your Mind,* "What we repeatedly think about and where we focus our attention is what we neurologically become."[2]

Just as when a gardener turns over the earth to aerate the soil and make it more hospitable to growth, I believe that to create conscious change we must "aerate"—bring focus and intention to—the suppressed aspects of our psyches. Doing so brings Heavenly awareness to mingle with Earthly density.

As you internalize the essence of the Law, *Circles Open into Spirals,* you will become more conscious of past influences that skew your perceptions and keep you stuck in closed circular patterns or downward spirals. Then you can envision more clearly how, within the context of changing cycles, to expand your learning and fulfill your potential.

Human Aspect of the Earth Triad: *Integrity Activates Change*

Within the context of the human aspect of the Earth triad, we must turn the Law from the Heaven realm into a workable Principle that functions within the natural cycles of human life. The primary lesson of *Integrity Activates Change* is that to truly move into a co-creative relationship with our Source, there is nothing that has happened or will happen in our lives that does not provide valuable information for growth and empowerment. The old adage "Learn from your mistakes" is only the beginning. As we shift away from old patterns of perception with their resulting behavior, we can discover how to integrate our experiences in new ways so that our "shit" can become fertilizer. As medical intuitive and author Carolyn Myss says, "Life is essentially a learning experience. Every situation, challenge and relationship contains some message worth learning or teaching to others."[3]

The task of the Human Principle—applying the Law for turning circles into spirals—is not easy. As I have stated earlier, in Western culture we attempt to think and act in linear ways. We're conditioned to try to eliminate the cycles and press on in a straight line upward and outward. Of course, since we *can't* stop the cyclical nature of experience, we interpret any part of a cycle that seems to go backward as failure. The task of applying an open mind and heart to all phases of our cycles can seems terrifying, not merely daunting. To keep the kind of integrity required to create transformational change may, at times, even seem to be impossible.

In an article published in *The Sun* called "The Blessing is Next To the Wound," Diane Lefer interviews Hector Aristizábal, a human rights activist, psychologist and actor-director who was severely tortured in Colombia, his country of origin, for owning "subversive" literature. Currently counseling others who have been tortured, Aristizábal says:

> Those of us who've been tortured need to see it as simply one more event in our lives, not a defining characteristic of who we are. And any time you go through a difficult ordeal, it can awaken inner resources. Instead of being a victim, each person can learn the lesson his or her spirit needs to learn.... For a long time, during the dirty war in Colombia, when my friends were being shot dead all around me, my goal was just to survive. But after I was tortured, my goal changed. It was not just to survive, but to live a meaningful life. Sometimes, in the ordeal, we find the seeds of our identity.[4]

The Principle, *Integrity Activates Change*, affirms that we cannot have integrity without integrating *all* that life has brought us, accepting and working even with events of unimaginable pain, whether or not those events happened because of conscious choices. When we do that essential work, we are able to move to a new level of awareness and personal power that is alchemical—that transforms straw into gold. The joy which then fuels our life is infinite.

Earth Aspect of the Earth Triad: *Allow Alchemy*

Here in this body are the sacred rivers: here are the sun and moon as well as all the pilgrimage places... I have not encountered another temple as blissful as my own body.
— *Saraha*

The Practice of the Earth triad, *Allow Alchemy*, provides practical tools for putting to use all that comes to us, be it easeful or challenging. Our physical bodies carry cellular memories, constricting and expanding according to past experiences and associations—patterns of reaction carried unconsciously though the brain's neurotransmitters and neuropeptides. When we infuse our bodies with *consciousness*, we become what Deepak Chopra refers to as "light beings," we become both the carriers and the conveyors of consciousness: Carriers in the sense that we have become aware of what we carry in our bodies and conveyors because we can share that awareness with others. Anything that happens in our lives eventually is composted, broken down into some form of energy, the ultimate self-ecology.

CHAPTER 9
The Cycles of Joy

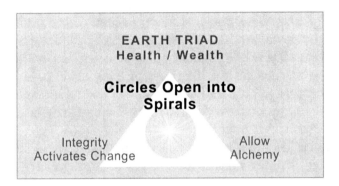

EARTH TRIAD
Health / Wealth

Circles Open into
Spirals

Integrity
Activates Change

Allow
Alchemy

Law of the Earth Triad

Healing
Happens in spirals,
In circles, yes
Circles that grow wider . . .
— *Monza Naff*

The third *Way of Joy* Law, *Circles Open into Spirals,* informs us that our lives are part of the greater natural world, which always functions in cycles. As beings within that world, our lives are also cyclical and will either unfold as closed circles within which we stagnate or open to spirals that allow us to most fully realize our potential. Whether conscious or unconscious, we make continual choices about whether to repeat or grow.

Circles Open into Spirals provides the universal concept that shines throughout the Earth triad. The inspiration that characterizes Heaven's expansive consciousness provides a context for the following questions in the Earth realm: If Source or the Divine manifests itself through us, what do we choose to create with that energy? What is the nature of evolution in our own lives, and how do we align with the natural world to foster optimal growth?

Caught in an Eddy

Nature is in constant motion, following cyclic patterns that describe the process of trans-formation.
— *Harriet Beinfield*

Tina, who had been feeling miserable and depressed for months, went on a hike hoping to find some solace in Nature. Coming upon a small creek, she sat down on a flat rock and gazed into the flowing water. Her eyes fell upon a leaf swirling around and around, trapped in a little eddy.

As she watched the leaf, Tina thought about her life. She had been feeling caught up in her own misery, sure she had no means of escape. Looking into the water, she realized she felt as trapped as the spinning leaf, as though she, too, had been caught up by a similar force. She wasn't happy with her career, felt stifled in the town where she was living and was feeling disconnected from her adult children, a son and daughter she had been very close to when they were young. She knew her husband, Bill, was getting sick of her attitude, which made her even more irritable. She was terrified that she would never be able to change her circumstances in any way that would really make a difference.

I believe that most of us feel caught in that eddy at different times, perhaps with a job, perhaps in continuing to be involved with partners who are remote or even abusive.

As these life patterns recur again and again, they begin to feel unchangeable, even inevitable. How many parents have found themselves using the same harsh tone and phrases with their child that they had experienced in their own youth and had promised themselves *they* would never say? It is as though they feel genetically pre-programmed to engage in the same dysfunctional communication their parents had before them as well as thwarted in their ability to parent differently.

When we examine the different dynamics operating in our lives, we will find many refrains from the past. Recently, my friend Jacquie complained to me about her partner. "I'm sick of always being taken for granted!" she declared. "He didn't even thank me when I went to his apartment and cleaned his oven for him. Why's it always like this with every guy I get involved with? Once the initial passion dies down, it's like we settle into being a boring married couple." Looking at her history of relationships, Jacquie was finding she was again experiencing a dynamic she didn't like or want. The intimacy she craved with a partner turned into a pattern she found deadening.

From a psychological perspective, we might find links from Jacquie's childhood, such as a parent who is the seed for her unconsciously expecting and drawing to herself a series of unappreciative partners. However, regardless of origin, when we find these patterns in our lives and don't pay attention to them, the cycles become closed circles that we're doomed to revisit again and again. We become stagnant in our inability, or unwillingness even, to allow optimism, let alone engage in creative problem-solving. So we allow our past to determine our future, as though we were putting ourselves through a karmic treadmill, repeating the same thing until we "get it right," as if we could.

We are unaware of how we are participating in creating self-fulfilling prophecies. We don't see the choices we make, be they conscious or unconscious, as leading to these patterns. Feeling powerless to change our lives translates into feeling victimized—by others, or even life itself. Then we often blame ourselves for being somehow inherently inadequate, damaging our self-esteem.

Perceiving Life as Linear: A Self-Fulfilling Process of Failure

What is it that keeps us so stuck? Once again, I believe, messages we've received in our Western culture block our evolution. One such belief is that life is supposed to be linear—we are born, grow up, and die—and whether we get what we want or not, we're supposed to "get over it" and move on. We're taught to see repeating trends as a failure to progress.

As I've gotten older, it has become ever more apparent to me that life is not linear. I think life lessons always seem to return in circular ways. I've found I may cycle many times through certain core issues, sometimes stumbling unaware, other times incorporating what I've learned. This cyclic pattern reminds me I am simply in accordance with the laws of the natural world. Neither our lives nor our healing actually proceed in a straight line.

Resistance to Self-Examination

Another behavior keeping us stuck in the eddy is a resistance to looking at whatever valuable information life recurrences offer, which is a resistance to life itself. This resistance to self-examination is, I believe, a direct offshoot of linear thinking, which gives us so many "failure" messages. We fear what we find could be worse than what we already know.

Take the example of Kevin, an adult man who had a hypercritical, demeaning and cruel mother. Kevin reacted to any feedback, constructive or not, as if an unjust authority were undermining him. He simply couldn't hear feedback unless it was 100% supportive. Because the emotional and cognitive associations he made whenever he received negative feedback were so tied to his mother, he always ended up believing he was being told he was inadequate and a failure.

Only if Kevin decided to do the inner work required through therapy, forgiveness, prayer or some other process of resolution could he create a new dynamic to break out of that dead-end loop. If he did that inner work, the energy bound up in a repeating circle of criticism/resistance and shame/blame could spiral open into a far wider range of responses to feedback where he no longer felt his very being at risk each time his actions or motives were challenged. It doesn't mean he would no longer receive criticism, even harsh feedback, ever again in his life. However, his perception of and response to that feedback would change dramatically.

When we resist feedback, I think we stunt our capacity for clear analysis of others and ourselves. The consequence is that we live in a world of denial and false hopes, where we block our own happiness and don't even know it.

Each time Jacquie started a new relationship, she'd think, "This time it'll be really different. He's so considerate, unlike the last guy." Wanting so much to believe in that difference, Jacquie may have missed cues to the contrary. When she reached a certain level of intimacy, she'd come to the painful realization that the dysfunction was happening again and her new partner was becoming less and less appreciative of her.

On the other hand, she might be with someone who actually *was* different, but when her buttons were pushed, she'd still conclude the new person was just the same as everyone else in her past. So Jacquie would miss an opportunity to have a healthier relationship and ask plaintively, "Why's this happening to me again? He seemed like such a great guy."

Although Jacquie tries to "move on," she can't. When she gets signals, either from a partner who actually does take her for granted or merely because she feels triggered even when her partner is *not* actually unappreciative, she sees herself as a victim of either her new partner or her own inability to attract the "right" person.

If she simply keeps changing partners without doing any inner work, her dismal choices appear to be to either carry on in misery or to collapse into despair. The attitude that we have only the no-win choice—to just "move on down the road" or become losers—is symbolic of what I would call a linear approach to life. If a relationship "fails" there's no use "looking back." We must just move on and try to find success in the future.

The Downward Spiral

Turning and turning . . .
Things fall apart;
the centre cannot hold
— W.B. Yeats

Circling around again and again through dysfunctional patterns, numb and resigned, muffles our sense of creativity, power, and ultimately spirit. When we get stuck in a no-win loop, we eventually become stagnant. In Taoist systems of healing, energy that ceases to flow is the primary cause of much disease and emotional pain. Just as a stagnant pond draws mosquitoes, negative thoughts buzz around with nagging persistence while our hearts are stung.

However, even when we circle in stagnation, nothing really stays the same. Stagnation ultimately leads to a downward spiral of increasing helplessness, fear, anger, self-doubt, and depression that deplete your energy. At this point, we move psychically into what I think of as an "inverted" spiral, where the center collapses and, like water going down a drain, the flow circles inward on itself, becoming ever more constricted.

The voices of the downward spiral are as seductive as a siren's call, enticing us to crash on the rocks of self-pity or vengeance: "Now *she'll* know what it feels like," "He'll be sorry," "Why does this always happen to me?" In this underworld kingdom, the victim mind-set is the ruler. The options here are few and all no-win. So how can we ever interrupt the loop and open that closed circle into a spiral that moves up and out instead of dragging our spirits down into the abyss?

Life Cycles and the Seasons

Nature moves in a continuously unfolding cycle of seasons, and there is no point at which its motion entirely stops.
— Ma Deva Padma

I think observing the cyclical patterns of nature can help us move away from linear thinking and recognize how growth is cyclical in human beings as well. Taoist philosophers consistently remind us to go to Nature to gain perspective and move into alignment with it. As Harriet Beinfield and Efrem Korngold say in *Between Heaven and Earth: A Guide to Chinese Medicine*, "Sustained by the power of Earth and transformed by the power of Heaven, humanity cannot be separated from Nature—we *are* Nature, manifest as people." Seeing ourselves as "Nature manifest as people,"[1] reminds us that we live in a cyclical world where our planet revolves around the sun in a cycle of day and night, where flowers and trees are born, die and reseed into new life, where seasons cycle through every year. Likewise, throughout our lives, I believe we too find ourselves in different "seasons" of life, death, and rebirth.[2]

Any event that recurs—happens in cycles—functions like a season. For example, a different "season" in a cycle could be times when you need to "let go" because of a death or other loss, or when you discover new things that inspire you. These could be occasions, such as spending time with your own parents or starting a new project or job. They could also be habitual emotional patterns, such as experiencing a block in your creative energy, or feeling overwhelmed by all that's on your plate. If we can learn to see any type of significant experience that occurs in cycles as a recurring season in our lives, we transform our own potential for growth.

Within each of these "seasons" are smaller cycles. Yet the cycles that repeat are not necessarily closed circles. One year the season of winter (larger cycle) might cycle through times of rainstorm with lightening and thunder, mild weather, or snow and sleet (smaller cycles). In the same way, while you might have a regular cycle of visiting your parents, where key issues are always stimulated, the "weather" might change from one time to the next, in terms of the ease or difficulty you have spending time with them.

I have one friend who struggles with chronic pain. Determined not to become a victim to her disability and its impact on her life, she wisely identifies the short cycles of her feelings and moods as they fluctuate from day to day as weather patterns. By looking at her varying internal responses to her pain as weather, she regards her feelings to be like transient clouds, storms, or tornados. As a result, she feels both comforted and empowered. She can better "weather" the weather.

Even with the variations in "weather" we can have different qualities of experience. We can lose our center, spiraling downward, or we can honor the seasons, knowing that their cyclical nature is part of our own process of transformation.

The Observer Self

When Tina reflected on that spinning leaf, she saw it as a mirror of her own life. Her flash of insight came to her Observer Self, a gift from the Heaven realm, as though she was observing her life in a detached and compassionate way from out in the cosmos. Whether she continues to circle in her own eddy or sets an intention how to change her life (Human realm) is now up to her.

Just as a stagnant pond needs air and movement to flow once more, the air (the breath of consciousness)—the yang energy of the Heaven realm—can break up the stagnation of our victim mentality—that old and familiar plaintive cry of "why me?"

When we recognize our lives as cyclical rather than linear, we can observe our patterns as we would observe nature, without judgment, blame, and shame. Then, it becomes possible to access the detached and compassionate view of the Observer, whose neutral perspective gives space for flashes of insight that can hit us with the force of lightning. Through the lens of the Observer, we can see things from a different perspective. This leads to a new level of understanding that can open the door to creative problem-solving.

Detached from our personal day-to-day dramas, the Observer can see our lives from a more holistic perspective. When we combine compassion for our choices, whatever they may be, and at the same time maintain the detachment to step back and hold a perspective of the whole picture, we are combining the wisdom of the Heaven realm with the love from the Human realm.

I believe it is absolutely crucial to draw upon the perspective of the Observer, especially when we feel stuck. This, I think, is the key to recognizing that everything we experience and manifest—all feelings, events, responses and so on—are part of a cycle. When we don't, we end up believing when we return to a certain dynamic that we haven't grown, can't change, or are somehow moving backward. Only when we become aware that we have simply arrived back at a certain point in our own cycle and can view our choices through a clearer lens do we find ways to unlock a closed circle and spiral into a new place.

As you practice drawing upon your Observer regularly, you will be better able to discern when there has been actual transformation, an opening of a circle into a spiral, and when there hasn't.

The Observer can also give us greater clarity in how we see others. Alicia was very concerned about her teenage son, Rodney, who had become very aggressive. When he was angry, Rodney developed the habit of taking an ax and going out into the woods behind the house and furiously chopping away at live trees, stripping away their bark. Following the advice of a therapist, Alicia began to set limits with Rodney to keep him from destroying the trees. One day, when she was with a friend, Alicia saw Rodney pick up an ax, throw a log on a stump and vigorously begin to chop it up. "See what I mean!" Alicia told her friend. "Nothing's really changed. Look at how angry he is. His energy is so intense." Her friend laughed and said, "Well, at least he's splitting wood. You'll have a good pile of kindling by the winter."

As you read this story, you might, like Alicia, remain focused on Rodney's aggressive behavior. But, as Alicia's friend observed, he was now channeling all of that intense energy he was feeling into something constructive, contributing to the winter stockpile of kindling rather than destroying the vitality and beauty of living trees. Rodney found that by channeling his anger differently he could "weather" his feelings during any "season" (cycle) when he felt intense frustration.

If his mother stays "stuck" in her old view and fails to notice this crucial change from destructive to constructive behavior coming out of Rodney's anger, it could impact how she treats him as well as how he sees himself. This attitude might slow down or ultimately derail the positive changes he is making.

The Pivot: From Carousel to Kundalini

A circle is closed and a spiral is open...You can't close a spiral. You can squish it like a Slinky, but it's still not closed.
— *Rachel Levine Chernoff*[3]

The moment we gain insight about our own self-defeating perpetuation of closed circles, we are at the pivot point for transformation. When we pivot, we turn ourselves around once more in a circle but this time towards growth and away from stagnation. Instead of losing our center, we expand from that pivot point into a widening spiral.

"Enough," Tina decided. "I don't want to be like this twirling leaf!" She stood up, picked up a nearby stick and thrust the tip of it into the current. The leaf made one more circle before dislodging from the eddy and joining the current's flow. Tina watched the leaf rush down the stream until it disappeared around a bend. She later told me that on her way home, she decided to look for a flyer she'd received about a *Way of Joy* Chi Kung Class and register. This was her first step, she later realized, in moving out of a state of mind where she felt victimized by her own choices.

Tina's pivot was spontaneous. Having accessed her Observer Self, she went seamlessly from insight (Heaven) to intention to create change (Human) to action (Earth). She symbolically freed the leaf as she wanted to free herself. Likewise, her decision to find the brochure was Human (intention), and her enrollment in the class was Earth (manifestation). Thus Tina's insight prompted two quickly spiraling cycles of intention and manifestation. The first, at the creek, followed the insight within moments, and the second, at home, within the hour. When we are sync, we move fluidly back and forth among Heaven, Human and Earth realms.

If we use everything that happens in our lives as food for change, we step off the merry-go-round of revisiting the same life lessons again and again. We transform knee-jerk reactions into heart-felt responses. As a result, the energy travels up and out, a Kundalini burst of consciousness that spirals up the backbone of our days.

Gargoyles at the Gate

Unfortunately, the kind of spontaneous insight and inspired change that Tina experienced at the creek doesn't happen as often as we might like. In fact, even awareness of seeing an old pattern come up again can prompt immobilizing fear and there is good reason why.

"Circling the drain," a metaphor sometimes used to describe someone who is dying, is apt here. There is something dying in this scenario—a way of believing, being and/or behaving, a dysfunctional pattern that, on some level, you are ready to flush away.

I believe every time we make a fundamental shift of consciousness that opens a circle into a spiral, we face a kind of death. Sensing this impending death, we move through a period of fear, facing our demons. Like gargoyles, these demons are the protectors of the gates of transition. When you feel yourself spiraling down, you might experience resistance, believing you have neither the means nor the courage to face what lies below.

Finding What's Useful in the Downward Spiral

With loss, descent, and death, there comes consciousness…There can be no renewal without death, without entropy, without regression.
— Clarissa Pinkola Estes

When you confront the gargoyles at the gate, you have three choices: to resist by running away and continue on the closed circle of the carousel, to continue downward into an inverted spiral, or to spiral up and out. If you are driven by fear, your choice will be unconscious, and more likely to block you from gaining insight.

Sometimes, though, it is only when we *do* spiral down to a more painful place that we get the impetus to change. This fits with the old saying about "hitting rock bottom" before coming back up, often talked about in 12-step programs. The risk is, some people hit rock bottom and stay there, unable or unwilling to climb back out of the abyss.

On the other hand, sometimes it is valuable to make a conscious decision to let yourself descend in a downward spiral, go into your resistance, doubt and fear. Here you *choose* to dive in, rather than being sucked down. Once there, you can explore that underground world as if you were walking around in a deep cavern and see what you discover there. You still have the "opportunity" at any point to call upon your Observer Self to help you look at what's below the surface so you can transform your cycle or you can seek the aid of a therapist, teacher, or spiritual guide. There are many opportunities in the shadows that allow a pivot to happen.

You need to be scrupulously honest with yourself during this process. Because the journey to the underground is the home of shame and blame, this is where we encounter the parts of ourselves we may be the most afraid to examine. But the voices there are crucial ones to listen to. When you do so, you will discover unacknowledged issues that you have not yet been willing to address, have disowned, or have lost hope about. Then the descent becomes the springboard to transformation. As the 33rd Chapter of the *Tao Te Ching* says, "To know others is wise; to know oneself, enlightened."

Making it Easier to Observe our Cycles and Pivot

As cycles and seasons go, there will always be another time to face one's demons in the depths. However, because accessing your Observer is a skill, I'd like to offer several ways to more fluidly move out of resistance into insight:

1. Use the First and Second Laws of Heaven to Access the Third

One of the fundamental ways to identify where you are in a cycle and pivot out of a stagnant pattern is to call upon the three Heaven Laws.

As the third Law, *Circles Open into Spirals* follows the other two— *Within Motion, Stillness; Within Stillness, Motion* and *Chi Moves in the Space Between*. Therefore, anytime things don't feel right, you can take a moment of mindfulness to attain the stillness inside of the motion of unending circles. Pause in whatever you are doing, stop thinking, trying to solve and resolve. As you breathe into your center, bring your attention to the movement of your inhalation and exhalation within that stillness.

Once you're balanced inside Stillness and Motion, you connect with the part of you who has the capacity to guide you to the Observer. Use this aspect to access the Law, *Chi Moves in the Space Between*. From a place of detached compassion, notice where there is stagnation, where energy is stuck or blocked, and where you perceive flow. Then, as you observe where in your beliefs, thoughts, feelings and actions energy is flowing and where it is not, you can opt to follow the flow.

Although she was not aware of any of these "Heaven Laws" at the time, Tina used these three concepts as a way to pivot. While sitting by the creek gazing at the leaf, she became attuned with the natural world around her and moved into a meditative state, where she balanced herself between stillness and motion. This allowed her chi to move and inspired an insight, which she then acted on to break open a closed circle.

Using the first and second Law of Heaven in order to access your Observer, you bring your conscious intention to your response to any situation. In so doing, you move out of a victim stance where you feel at the mercy of circumstances, and discover new ways to deal with old patterns and so utilize the third Law to pivot, opening circles into spirals.

2. Ask Curious Questions

When you break open a circle to create a spiral of understanding and inner progress, you are accessing the Divine within. As you breathe, finding the interweaving of motion and stillness and feeling the expansion of chi moving in the space between, you can ask genuinely curious questions of yourself, making it easier to access your own inner wisdom. You might ask, "When did I last experience this feeling? What approaches did I use in the past to cope with it? Did they work? If not, what can I do differently?"

If the last time you were in this place, you approached it differently and it did help you, then you can work to move out of any resistance that keeps you stuck in the old "orbit" and remember that new approach now. Often that grinding-to-a-halt feeling comes from doing the same thing again and again and seeing to your utter amazement that it does not lead to a different outcome.

Whether or not you have found a better way in the past, by using open questions you can summon your resources and creativity to find a new approach. Whether it is the "ultimate answer" or not, you will still break open a deadened pattern and gain new insight to lead you forward on your spiritual path.[4]

3. Express Insights and Create New Boundaries

Jacquie's relationship drama contains another example of how the pivot can function to bring new growth. In order to shift away from old habits, her first step would be to access the discerning eye of her Observer Self. By observing her own cycles, Jacquie can make different choices that will change her experience at the Human and Earth level. She can recognize that, regardless of the person she is with, the power to pivot is in her own hands. Jacquie can then identify her own patterns as well as more clearly name what she believes her partner needs to be accountable for. Using her creativity to act on new choices, she can break open the locked-in pattern of unsatisfying relationships and can renew her access to intimacy.

Primed with this perspective, Jacquie can then communicate differently with her partner about her past issues as well as what she'd like to do to change that pattern. She could say something like, "I realized you never thanked me for cleaning your oven, and it's been bothering me for a couple of reasons. One is that I wanted it to be a gift because you seemed so overwhelmed by the burnt smell that I thought it would make your life easier. When you didn't thank me, I wasn't really sure whether you appreciated it. The second thing comes from my own history. So many times when I get close, my partner seems to take me for granted and I end up resenting him. I don't want to recreate that with you, so I was hoping that we could look at it together, if you're willing."

As she and her partner talk, Jacquie has embarked on a pathway to greater intimacy. Or, if the partner is emotionally remote, she will recognize the signs soon enough to end the relationship before she becomes more emotionally invested.

Jacquie has clearly and honesty expressed her reactions and shared information about patterns shaped by her past. She can close with a prediction, letting her partner know that "if" he wants to look at this issue together with her, she would like that also. If he doesn't, she won't try to force it, but can create other boundaries around reciprocity. If she finds he's unable or unwilling to be reciprocal and appreciate her, she will then move on, but from a place of strength rather than failure.[5] Once she breaks this cyclical pattern in this way, she'll be much more likely to attract people to her who can be as responsive to her needs as she is to theirs.

Whether she chooses to pay attention like this or not, Jacquie is in a cycle. Her own choices will determine whether it will continue as a repeating pattern, reinforcing her negative beliefs, or pivot into a process that opens a spiral of awareness and potential for as yet untapped intimacy.

4. Pay Conscious Attention to Your Mood

Every day is the beginning of a cycle. What if, instead of turning on the television or radio, you tuned into your inner weather as you began the day? One friend told me she often woke up in the morning with a little wince as she anticipated the day ahead. After thinking about the theme of pivoting, she coined a humorous phrase to repeat before getting out of bed—"Drop *dread*, flow instead." This made her smile and shift out of a negative mindset before her feet hit the ground. Other people have told me when they wake up noticing a sense of anxiety about the day, they shift the internal weather by focusing on the things they are grateful for.

Whatever the time of day, rather than simply attempting to "overcome" those feelings of anxiety or dread, we can use them instead as a prompt to call upon our Observer for insight.

Gingerly balancing his coffee, bagel, and laptop briefcase, Manuel noticed that, as he had on recent Friday afternoons, he was feeling increasingly tense. As he passed by Carla, the receptionist, he noticed their supervisor, Bill, looking typically harried and talking urgently. Manuel glanced at the clock on Carla's desk—3:09 PM. Triggered by Bill's urgency, Manuel became more anxious, anticipating a last-minute request by Bill that he could not complete by 5:00. "Here we go again," he thought.

Manuel loved his work and, for the most part, had a good relationship with his colleagues. He held high standards for himself and was proud of what he had been able to accomplish for the small company. But he'd been filled increasingly with a familiar sense of dread. Every Friday afternoon for the last few weeks, Bill had appeared at his desk requesting that Manuel fulfill some assignment that needed urgent attention before Monday. Manuel ended up either staying in the office until late or, much to his wife's and kids' increasing frustration, he'd take the extra work home and do it over the weekend.

The more Manuel thought about it, the more irritable he became. He was as angry at himself for not believing he could prevent the inevitable flood of last-minute demands as he was at Bill for his insensitivity. Manuel knew he wasn't very good with boundaries. He'd come to realize there were times he had actually contributed to problems in his marriage and at work because he hadn't really learned how to be direct. The time had come, he thought with a groan, to try something new.

Manuel glanced at the photo of his family from that day at the ocean, then shut his eyes. He focused on his feet planted on the floor, and allowed the top of his head to rise up, imagining the gravitational pull of the earth below and the invitation of the sky above. He called upon his inner wisdom to guide him to make a change, any change, that would help him to pivot his expectation. Just as he opened his eyes, Bill rushed in with a large stack of documents.

"Manuel, I've got a project that needs to be finished so we can present it to the clients on Monday afternoon. Shouldn't be too hard. Thanks."

As Bill turned to go, Manuel took at deep breath, then asked him, "Bill, are you aware that this is the third time this month you've given me a task with an urgent deadline at the end of my work week?" Bill turned back slowly, frowned with a look of astonishment and asked, "I have? No, but why, is there a problem?"

"Yes, actually there is," Manuel said gently. "I'm aware of how much pressure you're under, and at the same time I know that earlier this week you already had a lot of this information you're asking me to complete now. I think when you're grappling with too many things at once, you end up asking me and others to wrap up loose ends at the last minute.

"Although it's OK with me to put in extra time occasionally, it's hard for me to understand why you waited 'til today to give me what you needed to complete the project. It makes my work incredibly pressured and I end up feeling I can't do an adequate job unless I give up my weekend. I care a lot about the quality of my work, and this job and the company, so it's meant that I've had to give up several weekends in a row with my family, which is hard on all of us. Plus this weekend is Angie's birthday.

"If you'd work to give me stuff earlier in the week, even if it's not all completely ready, then I'd not only feel less resentful, I'd also have time to do a more thorough job on the report."

Bill looked at him blankly for a moment, then shook his head. "You know, you're right," he sighed. "I do need to work on my flow charts, and I keep putting it off because there've been so many changes. I think when I get overwhelmed, I push everything aside until the last minute, and then I depend on you to pick up the slack. Look, I don't know if I can change this all at once, but I'd like to try. For today, would you put the rest of your projects aside, so that you could work on just this one piece until 5:00? I think that however much you do this afternoon would be enough to show the client we're making progress. Then, at the meeting on Monday, I'll map out the next piece of work so that the timing won't be so pressured. I'm grateful for all the extra hours you've put in lately, and I do want you to get out of here on time today."

Manuel sighed in relief, "I'll do as much as I can. And, hey, thanks."

As Bill left, Manuel added, " If you want, I could help you work on some flow charts next week."

"I bet you could," Bill teased, and they both laughed. Then he said, "Yeah, I think that's a great idea."

As a reader, you might feel some skepticism about this story. You might wonder how Manuel could be so articulate and calm about the issue when he felt so stressed about it. Or you might have thought it's not realistic for his manager to have responded so positively.

I'd like to review what happened with those questions in mind. Every Friday Manuel's body would tighten up in the early afternoon, giving him signals of anxiety even *before* he was aware he was expecting Bill to come in. Seeing Bill's agitation with Carla reinforced Manuel's distress. When his apprehension became a weekly reality, the cycle was cemented in his mind, and by staying *reactive* rather than responsive, he recreated the same pattern again and again.

Even though Manuel tried hard to *talk* himself out of his antipathy because he cared about his work, his feelings lodged "underground" in his body. It was not until he brought the light of his Observer Self's attention to those feelings that Manuel recognized his recurring dread as a *signal* that he was caught in the trap of a closed circle, a stagnating repetition of something destructive to him and to his family. Prompted by that insight, he created his own pivot point and then continued the pivot into an outward spiral by making a conscious choice to respond differently. That's when his situation changed. Manuel was no longer a victim to either his own fear of confrontation or his supervisor's stress and poor planning. He quickly manifested his insight and intention to change into what he needed, a new reality.

This kind of shift creates a change that is not only psychological and behavioral; it's also physical and energetic. In his book, *Evolve Your Brain: The Science of Changing Your Mind,* Joe Dispenza studies the physiology of the brain, the workings of the mind, the presence of consciousness or life force, and how they interact. Having healed himself from a serious back injury which leading surgeons and neurologists had determined would leave him paralyzed, Dispenza began to research people who had recovered from life-threatening illnesses despite the failed attempts of both allopathic and complementary (alternative) medicine. He found that across a range of age, gender, religion, race, sexual preference, educational status, class, fitness, and more, what these people had in common was their absolute belief that they had the capacity to heal themselves. He writes:

> It takes awareness and effort to break the cycle of a thinking process that has become unconscious. First, we need to step out of our routines so we can look at our lives. Through contemplation and self-reflection, we can become aware of unconscious scripts. Then we must observe these thoughts

without responding to them, so that they no longer initiate the automatic chemical responses that produce habitual behavior. Within all of us, we possess a level of self-awareness that can observe our thinking. We must learn how to be separate from these programs and when we do, we can willfully have dominion over them. In doing so, we are neurologically breaking apart thoughts that have become hardwired in our brain.[6]

When Manuel decided to not simply give in to his reactions and try something different, he actually did *change* his mind, and his brain rewired to create a new experience. When he made his pivot, he moved into his own flow, and information that was inside of him came out easily. The energetic shift in Manuel enabled him to speak without judgment and gave him a level of confidence that also impacted Bill, who was able to listen without getting defensive. In the process, Manuel not only changed a pattern for himself, he also changed his relationship with Bill. Able to gain new insight, Bill also had an opportunity to develop better management skills.

5. Intentionality and Activating Gratitude

In the previous chapter, *Cultivate Discernment*, I suggested ways to separate yourself from your narrative. I talked about stepping back not only to look at what you don't want, but also to make an assertion of what you *do* want. The proponents of the Law of Attraction talk about activating *gratitude*, which I believe has great power in helping us to pivot out of a closed circle or even a downward spiral. For instance, if I am feeling frustrated that once again I don't know what to say or do in a particular conflict, I can back away and observe the behavior, recognizing the pattern of self-doubt and subsequent frustration and anxiety.

At this point, it's possible to infuse a feeling of gratitude by calling upon the Observer Self and saying, "OK, slow down, I can look at this as a holding pattern, like an airplane circling around waiting to land, and appreciate this moment as giving me time to figure out what is going on."

The Law, *Circles Open into Spirals*, takes you back into the Heaven realm where as Observer you recognize core issues popping up, the appearance of habitual patterns of thinking, feeling, or behaving. This is the wise use of resistance, the possibility within the state of "Here we go again."

As long as our minds are filled with what is not working, there is no room for what might work instead. Conversely, embracing a sense of appreciation, wherever you are in your cycle, is profoundly empowering. It is an act of refusing to stay in a self-defeating pattern. When you express appreciation for *anything,* you spiral out of negativity into a more positive mind-set.

We can be grateful for our capacity to make decisions. We can be grateful, even in the midst of anguish, for our capacity to feel deeply. We can feel grateful to ourselves for taking a moment to do the inner work of noticing. What I am proposing is that we can actually be grateful for the opportunity to discern the nature and function of any current pattern and where we would like to go with it.

Conclusion: From Dead Ends to Evolution

Everything has to evolve…If it doesn't evolve, it stagnates.
— *John Steinbeck*

When we interrupt a habitual loop, we create the grounding to discover new potential, and so find ourselves making quantum growth spurts. Invoking the Law, Circles Open into Spirals grounds us in both inner and outer worlds that are in a constant state of change. You can:

Physically: Align your spine to let Heaven connect through your Human body to the Earth.

Emotionally: Activate gratitude, allow the flow of joy.

Mentally: Cultivate your capacity for discernment through using the Observer Self, the pivot, and the many gifts life presents in repeating patterns, so that everything becomes an opportunity to evolve.

Spiritually: Trust in the abundance of Source to direct how you want to work with repeating patterns.

As you deepen your Chi Kung practice, you will increasingly embody the realization that grounding means to be deeply connected to the earth in all of its cycles of transformation. Just as matter at its core is space, Earth at its core is change and growth. And we, creatures of the Earth, are evolutionary beings, spirals in the making.

CHAPTER 10
The Evolution of Joy

EARTH TRIAD
Health / Wealth

Circles Open into
Spirals

Integrity
Activates Change

Allow
Alchemy

Integrity Activates Change
Principle of the Earth Triad

You must be the change you wish to see in the world.
— *Mahatma Gandhi*

Integrity Activates Change explores the Human element of the Earth triad, where we look at how to effectively apply the perspective of the Law *Circles Open into Spirals* in your own life. As the Human aspect of each triad, the Principle always goes to the heart of the matter. At the heart of the matter in the Earth triad lie the following questions: Are you creating a life that is in alignment with your vision and your passion? More challenging, what do you do when you hit obstacles to your aspirations, when things appear to be harder than you expected? And even *more* challenging, how do you access joy to make choices when you are facing things that frighten, anger, discourage or demoralize you? That is, whether you initially see it as positive or negative, how do you pivot everything that happens so that it can be useful? The Earth triad is where you experience the real-life consequences of your choices.

With the first Principle, *Balance Brings Harmony*, you wholeheartedly embrace the apparent paradoxes in your life, the contradictions, being and doing, and so stay in harmony both internally and externally.

With the second Principle, *Boundaries Dissolve Barriers*, you define your boundaries, clarifying what makes you *you*, with an eye to what feeds you and what drains you. By letting go of either merging with another or becoming walled off, you are able to establish heart-felt connections with other people and with the world around you.

Now in the Earth realm with the third Principle, *Integrity Creates Change,* you are ready to move from embracing paradoxes and creating boundaries into the exciting realm of personal transformation. Following up on the Human triad, where you clarified what you want/don't want, believe/don't believe, here in the Earth realm you can harvest the results of that discernment process and do the nitty-gritty work of utilizing your creative potential. With this harvesting come the consequences of choices you have made along the way.

Weaving Straw into Gold

Creativity is our species' natural response to the challenges of human experience.
— Adriana Diaz

The magic of creating something extraordinary out of the ordinary may seem like a pipe dream, something way out of reach. However, I believe any time you've had an image of something you'd like to have happen in your life that actually did happen, you mastered, for that moment, the Earth realm of manifestation. You see a house in a magazine and you end up living in a home just like it. You feel a need for more support in your life and encounter a stranger at a diner, a person who becomes your best friend. Envisioning a delicious and healthful supper and then making it for yourself or your family is an act of manifestation. So is clearing out the clutter in your home and enjoying clarity around you, reading a bedtime story to a child and feeling the joy of fresh questions and a warm body snuggling close, or planting flowers in your garden and being nourished by the profusion of color and aroma. Actually, every time you rise out of bed to start the cycle of a new day, you are creating.

Manifestation Derailed

Manifestation happens constantly, but when we are stuck in situations we don't want or choose, we forget we have an innate ability to create change, even if it is simply by how we respond in a seemingly choice-less situation. We can manifest a train to our future goals. Likewise, we can manifest a train derailed. How we work our intention is a determining factor in how well we stay on track.

When Dispenza researched people who were threatened with an "incurable" illness, and found they shared an absolute belief in their capacity to heal themselves, he shed light on the power of conscious, disciplined intention. I have always been amazed at how many people who have achieved their potential at a world-class level—as artists, athletes, entrepreneurs, scientists, writers—describe knowing from a very young age what they would do. They too had extraordinarily strong intention and great follow-through. Without conscious intention, what we manifest too often fails to bring us what we really want and need in order to live deeply meaningful lives.

Manifesting What You Think You Want Doesn't Always Work

The first step in manifestation is to have a conscious vision (from the Heaven realm), then put out an intention of what we want (from the Human realm). At the same time, we can have a clear vision and work hard for it and still not be living a joyful life.

Even with all of the trappings of the American Dream, people often find the lives they have created are not giving them what they really want. In an article in the magazine, *Yoga + Joyful Living*, Pandit Rajmani Tigunait, author and spiritual head of the Himalayan Institute in Pennsylvania, describes his first journey to the United States. Tigunait came from an impoverished village in North India frequently beset by flood, drought, cholera and malaria. "Yet… immersed in a vibrant web of relationships with their family, their village and the natural world, they accepted their losses as part of life." Upon arriving in the United States, he was surprised to discover that, despite economic security, even wealth, many people were "unhappy… searching for an underlying sense of meaning and purpose in their lives. They saw themselves, not as part of a boundless continuum, but as individuals competing for… security in a troubled world.

"…They were full of fear and self-doubt and haunted by an underlying feeling of emptiness."[1]

It's Not Just What, But How

There are times when linear thinking is appropriate to our endeavors. For example, it is necessary when we are mapping out a series of tasks, doing scientific research, or analyzing the development of a new software program. Even here, the problem comes when we *exclude* the intuitive process as being of less value. For example, Newton was a brilliant linear thinker, but it was watching an apple fall that inspired his greater understanding of gravity.

I believe that our deeply internalized lesson about living life in a linear fashion is what derails us from manifesting what our hearts and souls need most. Linear thinking that prompts us to decide, "I'm going to marry that person," or "I'm going to get that promotion," or "I'm going to make sure my child gets into a good school."

When we name a goal and determine to use everything in our power to achieve it, there's no assurance that we will keep integrity in the process, or recognize along the way when something else is more important than that goal. We may push our child toward a nervous breakdown or a rebellion against academic achievement. We may end up with what looks like enviable success or the perfect mate while feeling absolutely hollow inside.

What Does it Take to Manifest in a Holistic Way?

I see manifestation as a spiritual journey—a coming home to your "best," most realized self. What you create with your life reflects your essential values, beliefs, talents and responses to circumstances as well as your capacity to make choices, commit to your own intention, and take a proactive approach to making things happen. How you go about that process is a combination of *how you "be"* and *what you do,* the balance of yin and yang. It requires first that you *be* rooted in the present moment and then that you accept and integrate whatever happens, whatever "the universe sends to you." It is not by attaining whatever you are striving for, but rather through the *process* of creating that you mature. You become, not "get" the prize. Does this mean you won't get any "prizes"? No, but the ones you get will bring deeper meaning to your life.

This takes discipline. Spiritual guide and poet Dr. Monza Naff identifies the root of the word *discipline* as disciple. She has reflected that the deeper meaning of *discipline,* commonly associated with work ethic, is actually a call to become a disciple of Self. I believe this is the meaning of "self-imposed discipline," as referenced by Ma Deva Padma, who says when "discipline is willingly taken on, self-imposed rather than endured because of external pressure or coercion, it will nourish your growth and deepen your maturity."[2]

The journey to come home to your most authentic, best self is both the path and the goal. We may even end up somewhere we never intended to go and realize it is just where we need to be. The question now is, How, even where, do we start?

Integrity: The Entire You

In practice, it all begins with the process of integration—integration of all aspects of our being and integration of the reality within and without. This process, in turn, begins with transforming ourselves. Only after we have collected the missing pieces of our private world and arranged them in a harmonious unity will our emptiness give way to a sense of deep, lasting fulfillment.
— Pandit Rajmani Tigunait

The basic premise behind the Principle, *Integrity Activates Change,* is that to create a life based in joy, you need to cultivate an ability to include all aspects of who you are and what you do. According to the Merriam-Webster Dictionary, the etymology of the word "integrity" derives from variations of the word *integrite* (meaning "entire) from Middle English, Middle French and Latin. Three parts of the definition are: 1) firm adherence to a code of especially moral or artistic values; 2) an unimpaired condition, soundness; and 3) the quality or state of being complete or undivided. I would like to look in order at each of these three definitions in relationship to the *Way of Joy* paradigm.

1. Your code of morals or values

To manifest a life in which you fully embrace your joy, you need to be in alignment with your values and convictions. This is true both internally—that is, how you process information through your psyche, mind and heart—and externally—how you put yourself out into the world, how you relate to others. Your values are embodied through the different roles you have—daughter/son, employer/employee, friend, or church/temple member and so on. To live where joy both fuels you and is fueled by you requires that you be connected to your own ethical code. Although those values may develop, even shift, as you accumulate experience and wisdom, to be in integrity you need to be in alignment with whatever ethics you feel strongly about. If you go against the grain of your own ethical beliefs, you lose not only a piece of your integrity or entirety, you lose yourself.

2. Soundness or unimpaired condition

Since the Earth realm is that of physical manifestation, integrity includes how you care for your own physical being, your *jing*, in the way structural integrity ensures the soundness of a building. The attention and support you give to your body as it ages is what keeps you grounded in the Earth realm. Chi Kung, especially the medical practices increasingly renowned for promoting vibrant health, are a superb way to maintain physical integrity.

On a more basic level, the simple act of physically aligning your posture is another entry point into your integrity. When you do, you access on a physical plane the wisdom from above and your strength from below. Sometimes, it's simply by straightening your spine that you can come back to your center and breath and so return to integrity.

Our essential integrity goes beyond physical soundness. In the past several decades science has uncovered more and more about the relationship between mind and body, a connection that Western culture has traditionally polarized. For example, research findings increasingly demonstrate that our cells retain early emotional shocks and traumas, that the bio-chemical structure of our bodies carry our feelings. Dr. Candace Pert, neuroscientist, researcher and author of the book, *Molecules of Emotion*, has said:

> For a long time, neuroscientists agreed that emotions are controlled by certain parts of the brain—the amygdala, hippocampus, and hypothalamus. This is a big, "neurocentric" assumption that I now think is either wrong or incomplete. But when I was a believer in the brain as the most important organ in the body, this assumption led me to do the right analysis in the lab for the wrong reason. Ultimately, it fueled my conviction that there are such things as molecules of emotion... Sigmund Freud would be delighted, because the idea that the body, in its totality, is also the unconscious mind, would be the molecular confirmation of his theories. Body and mind are simultaneous. [3]

The research of cellular biologist and author Dr. Bruce Lipton[4] and others shows that what a person *believes* can literally alter his/her genetic structure. This discovery supports the research of both Dispenza and Pert that the mind-body is one holistic entity.

3. The state of being complete or undivided

This final definition of integrity requires that all aspects of your being need to be integrated—physical, emotional, mental and spiritual. The integrity of the Earth realm, beyond your core values and the health of your physical body, also includes integrating what is happening "underground"—your ancestral heritage, your childhood, and your dreams from the unconscious world where your shadow side lives.

Integrity here means to listen to, honor, and integrate all of your internal voices—from your innocent child self, to your self-doubting inner critic—voices that rise up from below the surface unexpectedly. Regardless of what triggers you, these are the voices that stop you in your tracks. In fact, they are most likely to arise during some crucial point in your manifestation process.

When you have multiple voices clamoring in your head, you lose your sense of power, and the process of manifestation becomes dreary. When this happens, you end up creating what you never wanted, or you still feel unhappy, even when you achieve goals that would otherwise be fulfilling.

It's important to remember that bringing together different elements to make something new characterizes the essence of alchemy and the transformative process. Every part of yourself, whether you like that aspect or not, is contributing to the whole energetic system that makes you *you*. It's only when you are able to acknowledge and incorporate all parts of yourself that you become complete and undivided.

A Story of Transformation: From Victimhood to Empowerment

Michelle was seven months pregnant with her first child when her boyfriend, Merrill, took her to San Francisco for a surprise romantic stay at a bed and breakfast inn. The following morning, they walked to a little park in Hayes Valley where they used to spend time when they first began seeing one another. Here, thought Merrill, was the perfect place to propose to Michelle, the spot where a temporary temple had once stood and where they shared so many happy memories.

The morning air was still and the park quiet as they sat together on a bench, Merrill holding the ring that Michelle had designed, but not yet seen. He proposed. Michelle accepted. The moment was perfect. They sat together for a while looking at the beautiful ring and talking about their future together. They were enveloped in their own world of love and happy anticipation of the new family they were creating when a man carrying some kind of handmade sign marched up to them. The man began to talk, shocking them with his intrusion into this especially vulnerable moment, and ended with a demand for some money.

Michelle believed the man seemed fairly sane because he was speaking calmly. "We're in the middle of a special moment," she said. "So I'd appreciate it if you would please leave us so we can be alone together."

"I'm having a moment too!" the man retorted. "Are you pregnant?"

Knowing, at seven months, that the answer was obvious, Michelle and Merrill just looked at him, speechless.

"Well, I hope your baby dies!" His voice was calm, deliberate and as sharp as a knife. The curse barely off his lips, the man wheeled around and left them stunned.

It took several moments for the shock to wear off and for the man's words to sink in. Tears came to Michelle's eyes. This man had just uttered the worst words she could ever imagine hearing a man say to a pregnant woman. She felt as though his words had entered her very being and shaken her to the core. Terrified, she felt them resonating in her body. "Will his words pierce through me and hurt me and my baby?" she wondered anxiously. "What does it mean that this man approached us with such ugly energy right when we were feeling such love and happiness?"

Merrill, shaken himself, did his best to comfort her. "He's unconscious and doesn't know what he's saying. He can't hurt us," he soothed. But Michelle kept hearing his words—"I hope your baby dies!"—echoing inside herself.

Michelle wanted to throw off the curse, to be cleansed of his cruel words, to create a boundary to protect her and her child. Then she knew what she could do. She remembered a Chi Kung exercise she'd learned in a class she'd taken with me the year before at John F. Kennedy University. At the time Michelle had specifically asked me about how to create healthy energetic boundaries, and I'd recommended that she practice *Lotus Wafting* (see p. 245).

Michelle stood up and walked a small distance away from the bench. Taking a deep breath, she lifted her arms and began to practice the form, emanating energy that was simultaneously openhearted and protective. Merrill joined her and together, with intention, they sent out a prayer of love, including the man who had accosted them. They asked that he find "peace and a healthier, happier place to be."

Michelle related all this to me a week or so after the incident (and over a year since I had last seen her). I was profoundly moved by her inner power to pivot in this story. When I asked her if she remembered what she was feeling physically, she said when doing the *Lotus Wafting* Chi Kung form she felt both a clearing and a protection. She told me she felt as though the man's negative energy, a toxicity she had experienced as trying to creep into her, dissipated and left her body. She knew she and her baby were safe.

After the incident, Michelle and Merrill spent some time talking about how this experience symbolized what life might hold for them in the future. They spoke about how sometimes two very different worlds can just collide and have a huge impact and decided they wanted to be able to transform "whatever was thrown at them."

Just as they were discussing their future, a family walked past them and began playing together on a little jungle gym nearby. "It was amazing," Michelle later told me. "Right after experiencing that negative force and then doing the work to transform it, here came this family that looked so happy. It was like a vision for our own future." Merrill and Michelle walked over to the family and spent some time talking with the parents. By the time they left the park, they felt their love for one another and their hopes for their anticipated family had been reaffirmed.

I think this story is a profound example of how integrity activates change. Michelle moved astonishingly quickly from feeling like a victim into transforming and healing what had just happened. By choosing to practice *Lotus Wafting*, Michelle embraced all three meanings of *integrity*: being complete and undivided, ethical, and physically sound.

Michelle was able to access her Observer Self quickly and move out of any denial about the impact of the incident. First, she recognized her anxiety about her baby and the threat this negative energy might have on her pregnancy. Second, with her Chi Kung prayer, she made a choice to act in accordance with her own core value of love despite her shock. Third, she alchemized fear and worry into a state of personal empowerment. She and Merrill reinforced their *jing*, their physical strength, by clearly and intentionally running chi through their bodies with *Lotus Wafting*, a choice which enabled them to reclaim their power. The wave of energy that resulted rippled out and it is not a surprise to me that shortly afterward, they encountered a family who seemed to be an embodiment of their own future.

When Michelle and Merrill reclaimed their power, they interrupted a cycle of victim and perpetrator, activating a pivotal change that totally redirected their energy—transforming fear into love. As often happens, that wave of transformative energy also rippled out beyond that particular time and place. Michelle's story so inspired me that I told it to others. As I did so, I witnessed that energy become a kind of contagion of empowerment. As other people who heard Michelle's story began to remember ways in which they too, through staying in their own integrity, had alchemized painful obstacles into material for growth.

Accepting "What is... is"

I believe a fundamental step to achieving integrity is to have a clear picture of what is actually happening in one's life and accept the reality of it as a starting point, the clay to work with. Had Michelle not recognized the potential power of the man's attack, she might have just tried to "pass it off," while its toxicity continued to affect her. Ironically, had Michelle denied the impact of the aggressive psychic attack, she would have more likely become a victim to it.

Have you ever told a friend about a problem and they responded with advice about what they would, or you should, do, yet all you wanted was be witnessed and heard? Often, as we try to offer love and support to others, we rush in to "fix" things before acknowledging the reality of a situation. This keeps us in denial.

In Michelle's case, a friend might have said, "Oh, that man doesn't have any power to hurt you, just forget it," prompting her to feel silly for making such a big deal of it. She might then suppress her feelings. In the future, she might have become overprotective of her child, either from conscious fear of the man's "curse" or without conscious memory of what prompted her to parent that way.

Another aspect of denial is persisting in wishing something had "turned out differently." I often ask myself: 'How much time and energy do we as human beings waste staying stuck in the past, unable to be fully present with what is actually happening?' Staying stuck in the past also makes us feel like helpless victims.

Accepting "what is" means two things. The first, addressed already, is the need to move out of any denial, where you try to "rise above" what is not working for you. One of the many lessons I learned from Dr. Quinn is that when you feel ungrounded, merely recognizing and naming that fact is in itself grounding.

The second step is to release trying to control other people or circumstances. Had Michelle tried to control the man, she might have argued or tried to get him to take back what he said. Thinking we can control things outside ourselves is a form of "power over," and prompts resistance and power struggle, a losing battle that is another form of denial.

Moving into a state of acceptance means an unqualified "yes" to the present moment. This takes you into the flow that I believe is at the core of the Tao, where you are at one with the Now. The middle verse of Stephen Mitchell's interpretation of the twenty-third verse of Lao-tzu's *Tao Te Ching* reads:

> If you open yourself to the Tao,
> you are at one with the Tao

and you can embody it completely.
If you open yourself to insight,
you are at one with insight
and you can use it completely.
If you open yourself to loss,
you are at one with loss
and you can accept it completely.[5]

Acceptance, Not Submission

I want to be very clear that when I speak of accepting the reality of what is going on, I do not mean *submitting* to it. I do not mean "there's nothing you can do to change things so just buck up and deal with it." I mean something very different.

When I say to *accept*, I mean to take away any veils that keep you from seeing *what is* from one moment to the next. Only then will you be able to make clear choices about how you want to relate to the situation rather than getting stuck in a self-defeating and powerless mind-set such as "it is not supposed to be that way" or "it's just not fair."

Choosing to accept "reality" as it is in any given moment is not easy. The trap here is that the fantasy of "what should be" becomes more dominant in one's thinking than the opportunities embedded in "what is." For many people the idea of acceptance is so connected to "submitting" or "enduring" that they feel the choice to "accept" would result in even fewer choices than they already have.

Arthur suffered from chronic neuropathy in his legs. He had gone to several practitioners, both allopathic and complementary, to find solutions to his debilitating pain. Some were able to help and some not, but in general, his condition was getting worse. He felt his life was narrowing down around the pain. As his pain increased, he became not only frustrated with the ineffective treatments, but also angrily blamed himself for not taking adequate care of himself. He was stuck in a pattern where he not only suffered the consequences of his disability, he was also suffering over his suffering—that is, he was unconsciously compounding his problems by heaping self-blame on top of his very real physical condition.

Compare Arthur's response to that of a woman who, as she lay dying from a virulent and very painful form of cancer, told her companion she had discovered how to make room for her pain. She found if she allowed the pain to have space to *be*, she could open further to an even larger space where the pain was not. No longer trying to exert control over her suffering, her decision to accept "what is" allowed her to expand to a place where the entirety of her experience became far greater than the pain she was enduring.

I think that when we are faced with pain, as well as other kinds of difficult challenges, we tend to think that accepting the situation is the end of the road, a sign of giving up. But what we are truly giving up is the fantasy of "if only." Rather than the end of the road, acceptance is actually the beginning of the road—the first rather than the last step—because it leads us to a place where we can open the door to choose new options. Acceptance requires that you cultivate attentiveness, not just to what is wrong, but also to what is right, to what you feel grateful for. Instead of thrusting yourself into a state of scarcity, a mind-set that tells you there are not enough resources or possibilities, take the moment to breathe into how things *are*. Rather than limiting yourself to "either/or" thinking, move into "all/and." Once you do, you will be telling yourself the *whole* truth, which is another way of being in integrity.

The challenge here is to be in the present moment *just as it is* as part of the gift of being whole and alive—even when you are in extreme circumstances that bring you to your knees, when you don't know if you can take it anymore. There is *always* the possibility of transformation and a path back to your essence. Thus, to *accept* means to *surrender* in the Buddhist sense. Let go of thinking you have to control or even *can* control the outer world. When you do, you will have prepared the ground to alchemize the straw of loss and scarcity into the gold of maturing and enduring wisdom.

What if I Just *Can't* Accept? Constructive and Destructive Uses of Resistance

Resistance is one of the most difficult challenges we encounter on the "road of acceptance." You might say resistance is the shadow side of acceptance—they go hand in hand. In their book, *The Life We Are Given,* George Leonard and Michael Murphy, two of the founding figures of the human potential movement, write of resistance as a natural built-in response:

> Every one of us resists significant change, no matter whether it's for the worse or for the better. Our body, brain, and behavior have a built-in tendency to stay the same within rather narrow limits and to snap back when changed—and it's a very good thing they do. Just think about it: If your body temperature moved up or down by 10 percent, you'd be in big trouble. Same thing with your blood sugar level …This condition of

equilibrium, this resistance to change, is called homeostasis. It characterizes all self-regulating systems, from a bacterium to a frog to a human individual to a family to an organization to a whole culture. And it applies to psychological states and behavior as well as physical functioning. …Homeostasis …doesn't distinguish between what you would call change for the better and change for the worse. It resists *all* change…Still, change does occur—in individuals, families, organizations and whole cultures. Homeostats are reset, though the process might well cause a certain amount of anxiety, pain and upset.[6]

In the context of the Principle of *Integrity Activates Change,* resistance can be both destructive and constructive. Our resistance is destructive when it causes *more* suffering, when it functions as denial, a refusal to accept "what is." Refusing to "accept" has the same impact as refusing to hear feedback, which leads to stagnation.

On the other hand, you may find at times that your resistance is incredibly useful, even when it seems to hold you back, because, if you look at it more closely, it contains information you do not have readily available. Resistance can actually be a hidden part of your discernment that, like the friction of a tire against the pavement, moves you forward.

The Role of Resistance in Keeping Integrity with our Values

Resistance itself can be an essential tool that supports our integrity and all levels of our self-integration. For example, resisting oppression, racism, or other forms of social injustice is a way to keep integrity in terms of a moral code. And resistance training, such as isometrics or specific Chi Kung exercises, strengthens our bodies, reflecting integrity in the physical aspect. There are times you may find you are feeling resistant for a good reason. It is important not to talk yourself out of your resistance or to place value judgments on it too soon. First accept it, then discern if it is a form of denial, a cue to stop what you are doing, or an ethical position you want to hold. There is a saying, sometimes attributed to Fritz Perls, the founder of Gestalt therapy, that "fear is excitement without breath." Whenever you feel immobilized by your own fears and resistance, regardless of how they come to you, you can always take the opportunity to stop, trust the process, take that deep breath, and listen deeply. Jack Kornfield, Buddhist meditation teacher and author, writes:

We must inquire what aspect of this repeated pattern is asking for acceptance and compassion, and ask ourselves, 'Can I touch with love whatever I have closed my heart to?' This doesn't mean solving it or figuring it out—it is simply asking, 'What wants acceptance?' In difficult patterns of thought, emotion, or sensation, we must open to feel their full energy in our body, heart, and mind, however strongly they show themselves.[7]

What Is "Reality" and What Does It Mean to "Create" It?

Many practitioners of the Law of Attraction assert that everything that happens in our lives is ultimately a product of our thoughts and feelings—that we "create our own reality." I, too, have presented examples where people like Tina and Michelle made a "new reality" out of an existing one.

I agree with the fundamental principle behind the Law of Attraction—that each of us is, in essence, made up of energetic vibrations that resonate and interact with the world around us. When we tap into that awareness, marry it with our intention and actions, we have the capacity to create more with our lives than we might've previously imagined. I think that the most important gift of a movie like The Secret, or the work of those who espouse the Law of Attraction or the Power of Intention, and so on, is that this way of thinking empowers people to believe that they really can make choices that open up new realms of possibility, that they have the capacity to create profound transformation in their lives.

There's a directive embedded in the "you create your own reality" school of thinking that I believe can be very helpful. When something's happening that is painful or challenging, it's wise to place your focus on things that are already working well in your life. This reminds us that chi does indeed move in the space between, and when we focus on those openings, we find an increased flow of positive energy that both feeds us and emanates from us. The vibrations of our thoughts, actions and, most especially, emotions, resonate outward.

At the same time, I believe a hypothesis that says—We (all of us) create (cause to be) our own reality (every single thing that happens to us)—is an oversimplification. Putting an unbending emphasis on only "staying positive" contradicts any number of principles for integrating the Heaven, Human and Earth aspects of our lives. For example, this tenet doesn't include the value of resistance or going into a downward spiral as a potential tool for learning. Tenaciously holding on to an ever-positive attitude also denies us the option of delving into a wide range of feelings and working with them or of accepting our current reality without immediately trying to control it in some way. There is an old Taoist tale that goes something like this.

> There once was a farmer who had a beautiful mare. Many of his neighbors envied him, saying, "You are so lucky to have this horse." The farmer's response was always the same. "Maybe, maybe not. That is the way it is." One day the mare broke out of the corral and ran away. The villagers came to the farmer's house to sympathize. "What bad luck!" they exclaimed. The farmer answered, "Maybe, maybe not. That is the way it is." A few days later, the mare returned on her own, bringing with her a beautiful wild stallion. The neighbors gathered around the stable, praising the animals and rejoicing. "What good fortune you have!" "That is the way it is," replied the farmer. The following day, the farmer's son climbed up on the stallion, intending to tame it. The stallion reared and threw the son off, breaking his leg. As the news traveled, the villagers gathered around to express their sympathy and regret. Again, the farmer replied, "That is the way it is." Meanwhile, there was a war raging. A troupe of military men came to the village and conscripted all of the young men except for the farmer's son with the broken leg. All of them were killed in battle shortly after. Again the villagers were amazed by the farmer's good luck. "Maybe, maybe not," he said.

The farmer had the wisdom to recognize that what appears as good luck may not always be; and what appears as bad luck may in fact turn out to be very fortuitous. Most of all, the farmer had the ability to accept "what is" and go with it.

Yet another problem I see with the belief that "we are the sole creators of our own reality" is that people end up feeling blamed, either by themselves, like Arthur who was suffering from neuropathy, or by others for not attracting the "right" thing. I've seen many instances where, when something "bad" happened, people ended up back in that linear place of feeling like a failure if a certain goal was not achieved. They were angry at themselves, either because they didn't attract what they set out to, or worse, they attracted something negative.

I have seen proponents of this world-view unwittingly place painful and unjust blame on those who have experienced deep misfortune. When people conclude that everything that happens is under their domain and control, or will just happen only by "thinking positive thoughts," it becomes a kind of magical thinking or moral superiority.

The inspiring journey of Treya Killam Wilber as she lived and died with cancer is described eloquently in the book, *Grace and Grit: Spirituality and Healing in the Life and Death of Treya Killam Wilber.* Compiled by her husband, the well-known philosopher, Ken Wilber, this moving account includes much of Treya's own words, including an article—"What Kind of Help Really Helps"—published in several periodicals while she was still alive. This brilliantly incisive essay examines her own thoughts on the subject of "you create your own reality" and its impact on her. She wrote:

> I'm certain that I played a role on my becoming ill, a role that was mostly unconscious and unintentional, and I know that I play a large role, this one very conscious and intentional, in getting well and staying well…. I am also very aware of the many other factors which are largely beyond my conscious or unconscious control. We are all, thankfully, part of a much larger whole. I like being aware of this, even though it means I have less control. We are all too interconnected… life is too wonderfully complex… for a simple statement like "you create your own reality" to be simply true. A belief that I control or create my own reality actually attempts to rip me out of the rich, complex, mysterious, and supportive context of my life. It attempts, in the name of control, to deny the web of relationships which nurtures me and each of us daily. As a correction to the belief that we are at the mercy of larger forces or that illness is due to external agents only, this idea that we create our own reality and therefore our own illnesses is important and necessary. But it goes too far. It is an overreaction, based on an oversimplification. I have come to feel that the extreme form of this belief negates what is helpful about it, that it is too often used in a narrow-minded, narcissistic, divisive, and dangerous way.[8]

I agree with Treya Killan Wilber that this egocentric approach to life denies the interplay and influence of different and still-mysterious energetic forces. What constitutes a vibrational frequency is a complex combination of factors. Speaking about her thoughts regarding the Law of Attraction in an online interview, scholar and philosopher Jean Houston said:

We are part of a natural system. The inherent ability of natural systems is to spontaneously form new patterns of order, meaning that the future of any system—the future of ourselves—is always marked by novelty and surprise, not by programmed blueprints or wish-fulfilling, however intentional they may be. We can have intentions but (we also need) to know that the universe is working through us as "God's stuff incarnated through the lens of space and time," (which) is also going to provide us with chronic novelty, spontaneity, despair.

Our personal journey of manifestation is always coupled with mystery that is beyond our individual control. Or, as Dr. Quinn once put it, "Sometimes flowers just get stepped on."

For me, a far more interesting question is *how do you respond* to whatever is occurring? Rather than saying you totally create your own reality, I would prefer to say that you create how you *respond* to and thus *affect* your reality. The ways in which you choose to respond to any given situation colors your perspective. This in turn influences how you *experience* your reality. Then, because your subjective experience is different, you can also say that your reality is different. So, depending on the nature of your response, you *have* changed your reality.

So the bottom-line question for me is not whether or not we create our own reality, but how we *receive* and *respond to* whatever occurs. When something happens in your life and you transform it into a means for growth—even with particularly painful situations like the death of a loved one, undergoing a chronic illness, and so on—rather than trying to evaluate whether you have done a good or poor job of attracting it—it seems to me the real work is how to hold the stance of accepting, even welcoming, all that happens as food for spiritual/personal growth and development. I am *not* saying I think we should all rejoice when we feel pain and suffering. However, I *am* suggesting that you allow the present moment, whatever it is, to be a contribution in some way to the greater whole of your life.

Your choices to respond to adversity in ways that reflect your integrity not only influence your well-being, but also invite the spaciousness of the Heaven realm, through the eye of the Observer, to enter into the density of life's biggest challenges. Then it is possible for you to experience even the greatest pain in a way that does not feel oppressive or make you feel like a victim. By keeping the channels open, you can discover how you might use those obstacles either for information or redirection of your chi.

When you respond to difficult challenges in a new way, you spiral up and out of any expected or unchanging view of circumstances. To me, this is true change—even transformation—the result of which is a spiral of infinite possibilities. By accepting "what is" and managing the power of our own intentions and actions, we can live fully in our integrity, active participants with the universe in the co-creation of our reality.

Power and Integrity

I would like to finish this chapter with an autobiographical story. I have included it because it recounts an experience that opened me to a new level of understanding of how chi works and galvanized my own journey, both personally and professionally.

In the 1970s I spent time in France studying mime with Etienne Decroux at the recommendation of Marcel Marceau. I loved living in France and had a great desire to return and travel more in Europe. A decade later, after starting a women's theater company called Common Threads, I fulfilled my dream. In 1985, our company did a six-month tour in Europe.

It was during this trip that I went with Helga, my German friend, to visit the martial arts teacher she'd told me about who performed extraordinary feats. In the early seventies, I had seen films and demonstrations of Tai Chi and Chi Kung prowess that had impressed me. While I wasn't certain I would see something more extraordinary than what I'd already witnessed, I was intrigued, so I agreed to go. Several members of the troupe went with me, having received permission to come as visitors to the dojo. An abbreviated description of key episodes follows.

A Close Encounter

I look around the large dojo with interest and see our host, Wolfgang, about medium height, with dark hair tangled around his face. "He doesn't look very fit," I think doubtfully, as he watches his 30 students drift about the space, practicing a walking form. All of them are wan, expressionless, as they glide one foot down onto the floor then another. They almost seem to be sleepwalking except for a kind of wariness around their eyes."

I glance at my companions who watch the scene with varying degrees of fascination. My solar plexus tightens, it all seems so unreal. It reminds me of horror movies about zombies from my 50s childhood. "Don't be silly," I reassure myself. "Helga says he's really quite exceptional. Don't be so narrow-minded."

I watch Wolfgang engage in a push hands session with a young, pasty-faced man in his late twenties. As I watch Wolfgang's hand pass what looks to be six inches from the young man's face, the man's head snaps back, and I watch in amazement as his eye begins to swell. As they continue to move back and forth, welts appear all over the man's face, and he's having a hard time even keeping his arms up. Yet Wolfgang continues to make no contact, sweeping his hands at a distance from the boy's face and body as the bruises continue to emerge. Suddenly Wolfgang stops with a snort. The young man turns away, head bowed.

Wolfgang turns to us. "I will show you something else." He shouts out a command. The group circles around him. A well-toned martial artist, his taut face belying his loosely relaxed stance, stands in front of Wolfgang, who nods. The man approaches cautiously, then Wolfgang snaps out a demand. The man takes a deep breath and suddenly throws a punch toward's Wolfgang face. His tight fist seems to freeze in mid air a few inches from contact with Wolfgang's nose. The man frowns. Rolling up his sleeves, Wolfgang taunts him, jabbing out what appear to be directions. The man yanks himself back and then charges forward again, with a thrusting uppercut to Wolfgang's jaw. With a ghost of a smirk on the corners of his mouth and hands loose at his sides, Wolfgang casually raises his leg up into the air in front of him, foot flexed towards his opponent. I notice his leg doesn't extend fully as in a kick. I'm not particularly impressed by his technique until I see that, apparently without making contact, the young man bounces back as though he has been pushed, and is caught by a couple of solemn-faced men behind him.

Wolfgang grunts out a word, and the student heaves himself up once again and runs full force towards Wolfgang. I think I see an almost imperceptible shift or twitch in Wolfgang's spine. This time, the young man's limp body flies across the room and slams up against the wall behind him. Again, at Wolfgang's command, he wobbles up to standing, then charges, only to be flung back once more, arms flailing, by some invisible force.

This action is repeated over and over until, at last, Wolfgang makes another request and his opponent staggers away to join the circle of students. Suddenly, all forty men and women rush towards Wolfgang, fists raised. He stands planted in the center. Again I think I notice a very slight motion in his back. The direction of the people around him changes abruptly, as though they've hit some invisible barrier, and they begin to stumble clockwise around him, arms reaching out as though to stop the momentum and maintain balance. They look like rag dolls caught in some immense centrifugal force until he raises his arms and they break away in different directions.

A women introduces herself as Elke and tells me what a great man Wolfgang is, what a vision for society he has, how he understands the human condition. Elke tells us that Wolfgang's reputation has been spreading, that there are so many people who would like to come to be a part of his movement.

My mind tries to grasp what is not conceivable, that my entire sense of reality is dissolving. I don't know what to believe or not to believe anymore. "If what I've seen with my own eyes is real, then anything I can imagine may actually be possible and exist in some realm," I think. I feel as though I'm in some "episode of the Twilight Zone" or an implausible sci-fi novel. Yet I speculate on what this realization might mean in terms of politics, social change, even the survival of the planet. If anything that I can imagine might actually be real, the possibility of creative solutions is limitless.

Wolfgang enters the room and the murmuring stops. Helga tells him that I've been practicing tai chi for many years. "Ah so," he says. "But it is limited. It gives an illusion of yin/yang. Yin and Yang are not separate, it is all the same." He taps his teeth and says with a sardonic grin, "We're all the same."

After Wolfgang leaves, Helga looks at us, "Not everyone gets to see that kind of demonstration. He's given you a great honor." My thoughts about spending more time with him continue to fluctuate between curiosity and dread. One member of my acting troupe didn't even want to leave, so impressed was she with how Wolfgang's powers might be used for good ends.

My mind begins to spin. Change the world? Yes, we need to, but why do I feel so horrified? I want to run screaming at the very thought of staying much longer, let alone coming back. He is dangerous. I can taste it. But what if I'm wrong? What if there is a way to harness this power?

Back in the dojo, shortly before it was time to leave, Wolfgang stretches out his hand toward me and asks if I want to push hands. The air suddenly feels thicker as I slowly rise. As I move toward him, I recall the demonstration yesterday. Will I become another platform for him to assert his superiority? At the same time, I love to push hands and feel curiously unafraid, eager even, to experience the invisible force that I had seen in action. What will it feel like in my own body?

I think that he is talking as he places his hand on my wrist. "Don't let him know you're nervous, smile at him," I think, letting go of the breath I have been holding. We begin to push hands, back and forth, gentle, easy, exploring. This practice feels effortless to me, familiar like breathing. I begin to feel exhilarated, at one with him. "This is fun," I think. "Like dancing. Relax, relax deeper. Focus, pay attention." It becomes less clear who is pushing, who is responding. Our wrists seem glued together as we dip and rise. I believe that the dance is mutual, except that a dim part of me notices that he is the one doing all of the leading, that actually I am being led around the room, that my will is dissolving. But it doesn't seem to matter. It feels like our beings are merged, that the loss of my will holds a certain kind of ecstasy. Time disappears.

Like a lightning bolt out of nowhere, he strikes me between the eyebrows with his palm heel. It happens so fast I don't see his hand coming. Shocked, my mind reels. Physically it feels as though my face is a rubber mask that has been forced inside out and immediately pops out again. It is the oddest sensation I've ever had. Not exactly painful, but shocking, electrifying.

Stunned, I notice that he has separated from me and is walking towards the others. Then my awareness of all else disappears as I rediscover my face.

Conclusion: Defining Mastery

Sometimes, in the ordeal, we find the seeds of our identity.
— *Hector Aristizábal*

My memory after that time with Wolfgang is dim. I do remember that when we walked out of the dojo, we were all were dazed, in shock. As our van pulled out of the parking lot, one of us, then another, began to talk, giving ourselves a reality check to see if what we had witnessed had actually happened. Astonished to hear my description of my push hands experience, they told me that the strike between my eyebrows had looked like slow motion.

When I finally returned to the U.S., I got together with Khaleghl and described what had happened. She too was disgusted by this demonstration of abuse of power, but gently suggested, "It may have been your higher guidance that interacted with a higher source of his that caused him to strike you in your sixth chakra in order to open and awaken it."

This re-framing of an experience that I might have otherwise suppressed because it was too extraordinary, demoralizing, or terrifying prompted me to a new level of learning. I don't believe Wolfgang consciously intended to help me in any way, but, rather, wanted to demonstrate his ability to dominate me. But as time passed, I realized that my intuitive ability had indeed been sharpened. In fact, whether or not Wolfgang's higher self was at work here, my own guidance led me to use this experience in ways that would promote my growth.

Ever since the early Taoist immortals first went on a quest to discover the secrets of longevity, many others have attained the capacity to do extraordinary things. They demonstrate that, when humans harness and develop chi, anything is possible. The unexpected and boundless abilities of chi masters can inspire us, wake us up to vast *possibilities*, our own unlimited *potential* and infinite *power*.

My time at Wolfgang's school expanded both my awe and my humility about what can be attained through the cultivation of chi. But like a splash of cold water, it awakened me to examine at a deeper level the relationship between power and ethics. I'd been immersed for two days in an environment where power was being used to abuse and control people, to drain rather than share life force. It became crystal clear to me that despite how dangerous such use of power is, it was also very seductive to the people there. At that point, I recognized that a single focus of developing and mastering my own chi was no longer sufficient.

Having experienced on a cellular level the impact of Wolfgang's strike, my first reaction was to feel ashamed or powerless in the face of his vast abilities, but I realized I needed to transcend those feelings and redefine for myself the elements of true "mastery." My own definition of mastery has evolved to include not just *what* a master is able to do, but *how* he or she chooses to use those skills. Mastery requires integrity.

Integrating and expanding on my experience with Wolfgang exemplifies the Earth realm Principle, *Integrity Creates Change*. What I learned during that time is at the heart of what was to become a profound life change, an alchemy that has, in part, forged who I am today. For me to come to integrity, I had to 1) re-evaluate and live my core values, 2) strengthen my chi practices, and 3) integrate all of my abilities—physical, emotional, mental and spiritual. I have dedicated much of my life's work to building upon this renewed vision of mastery, which I see as an unfolding process.

What I suspected then, and am now convinced of, is that the most thrilling result of chi cultivation—true mastery—is becoming a "disciple of self." This shifts the expression of power from adversarial to integrative, from "power over" to "power within." I believe with all my heart that when you work to cultivate the "power within" yourself, you bring yourself home to center. When we desire "power over," we are motivated by fear or the attempt to conquer fear. When we cultivate "power within," we are inspired by Love, a joyful embrace of our wholeness. To develop power within requires that you accept and integrate all of who you are, align with Source, trust the essential qualities of your nature and bring forth your gifts.

Embodying this state of being through working your chi not only reinforces you, it causes an energetic ripple that resonates both inside of you and in the world around you.

I love to imagine a world where every person is called to live out his or her greatest talents, embody the soul's essence, honor the diverse gifts of others, and in so doing feel an interconnectedness, what Thich Nhat Hahn calls "inter-being" with all-that-is. As I see it, there could be no more wondrous achievement, no more profound mastery. This would indeed be the unending Source of creation that is the Earth realm.

The Way of Joy

CHAPTER 11

The Acceptance of Joy

```
                    EARTH TRIAD
                   Health / Wealth

                   Circles Open into
                        Spirals


        Integrity                      Allow
   Activates Change                  Alchemy
```

Allow Alchemy
The Practice of the Earth Triad

Hospitality is the fundamental virtue of the soil. It makes room. It shares.
It neutralizes poisons. And so it heals.
—William Bryant Logan

As I stand beside the long path of glowing orange-red coals, my entire body begins to shake. "I can't," I think, panicked. "I just don't think I can do it."

The Bay Area evening temperature is typically cool and damp, but I know the trembling I am experiencing is not because of the weather, at least not outside.

For several months before this moment I had been thinking on and off about what it might be like to do a firewalk, a ritual practiced for centuries and across world cultures in which participants walk barefoot over a bed of hot coals. While I wasn't exactly sure what drew me to want to do it, I had the vague sense that I had come to a point in my personal Chi Kung practice where I was curious to see how I might use my chi with that kind of challenge. I still remember the day when I decided if I ever heard of a firewalk in my area, I'd do it. Still, I felt safe in the assumption that day would probably never come. The very next morning, to my

disbelief and dismay, I received a workshop announcement in the mail
from someone I had never heard of, Georgeanne Johnson. It said that she
would be leading a firewalk near my home that very next weekend. It
seemed like the universe, in its infinite humor and wisdom, was going to
put me to the test. Who was I to refuse? Trying not to think about it too
much, I took a deep breath and mailed off my registration.

A large group of about thirty or forty people gathered, and the
workshop began early in the afternoon with each of us thinking about and
naming our intentions. Some were veteran firewalkers, while others, like
myself, were complete novices.

That evening, we went outside and built a huge bonfire. As it flared
into a full blaze, I began to feel all of my doubts and fears crowding my
throat. The smoke from the high flames burned my eyes, and I backed
away with not much in my mind except "What the hell was I thinking?"

The workshop leader brought us back inside and took us through a
process of listening to and facing our fears, then led meditations and reflections that allowed each individual to listen deeply to her own counsel. As
we prepared to go back outside and rake the coals into a long path, the
leader encouraged us to listen to our bodies, to wait until we were
absolutely certain before we walked onto the coals.

"It's really important to listen to your fear, to honor it and then use
it. Don't push it away." She ended by telling us. "Also know that it sometimes takes more courage to decide not to walk than to walk. If you do
decide to walk, it is important to let the fear be fully present and allow it
to transmute into pure energy." I was moved by the level of support within
the group and the belief that whatever choice each one of us made would
be the "right" one.

"I don't know if I'll be able to do this," I think stumbling back a step
as though pushed by the heat emanating from the fiery path of coals. Shiv-
ering with fear, I bow my head, accepting in a deep way that I do not
require anything of myself other than to stay present, to feel the fear and
not interpret it or decide anything. One woman after another, each in her
own timing, takes a step onto the fiery hot path and begins to cross. On the
sidelines, the rest of us raise our voices, offering vocal and energetic support
as the next one prepares herself. There are some who, when they get to
the head of the line, shake their heads, and move to the side, knowing that
the time is not ripe.

My teeth are chattering. Again I try to reassure myself, "I can always
choose not to walk, no shame." Nevertheless, as if in a dream, I move to
the line of women ready to walk. As I get closer to the head of the line, my

shaking increases, but my thoughts slow down. "What if I could just raise my energy to that of fire?" I wonder. "What if my shaking was the same, an embodiment of the shimmering of the flames?" As I look across the long path of steaming hot coals, I envision that I'm walking with confidence towards my future. "I want to honor the information that has been given to me and share my work with more and more confidence, ease and wisdom," I acknowledge quietly. By the time I step onto the coals, I am ready, my doubts gone. My spirit lifts as I stride purposefully to the far end of the red-hot coals which, crunching below my feet, do not burn me.

Firewalking was, for me, a primal experience with the transmutation of fear. In a ritual in which I was encouraged simply to permit my fear to be there—allow it to course through my body—without trying either to conquer or deny it, I learned how to be with all of what I was feeling in a very visceral way and so alchemize those feelings into pure energy. This process of allowing, where I was not actually *doing* anything but staying present with my state of *being*, produced a transformation in my body. As I let myself be with physical terror, a shift happened, and, as my body shook, I experienced a profound release. As a result, it seemed the heat of my own energy rose up to match that of the red hot coals, and my chi became one with the chi of the fire. Then, as I aligned with my higher purpose—committing more deeply to my own spiritual path—I believe I activated a deeper alchemy in my whole being.

As we saw in the previous chapter, different types of resistance, especially fear, are a common companion on the road to empowerment. As you move from inspiration and intention into form, unaddressed shadow sides must be dealt with to complete the manifestation of anything important. In the Practice, *Allow Alchemy*, the Earth aspect of the Earth triad, you'll often find yourself facing all of those feelings you haven't been willing to face so far. Like the final stages of birth, the manifestation process—the embodiment of Heaven's vision and Human intention—can be hard labor. When whatever you are creating is ready to be born, you need to summon your resolve to give a final push. At the same time, birthing has its own momentum, so the task requires both surrender and enormous stamina, not unlike the release I experienced as I stepped onto the bed of hot coals.

In the Practice for the Heaven triad, *Embrace Wholeness,* we focused on accepting polarities. With the Practice of *Cultivating Discernment* in the Human triad, we focused on grounding our ability to determine what we need from what distracts us, blocks us, or otherwise hurts us. In the Earth triad, the final Practice, *Allow Alchemy,* we will take a final step to make everything in our lives, even our most difficult feelings, of use.

When Resistance Gets Stronger

Our greatest fear is not that we are inadequate, but that we are powerful beyond measure.
— *Marianne Williamson*

One thing that makes the Earth realm so difficult is that in this final stage of manifestation we encounter any of the remnants of resistance we have so far been able to avoid or circumvent. When we do, we must journey into the underground of the unconscious mind to address whatever may still be there that has held us back from reclaiming our power, issues that have kept us from being able to fully experience our enthusiasm for life.

Often, just as we're about to flower, obstacles seem to emerge from the underworld of the unconscious—fear, shame, self-blame, self-doubt, mistrust, anxiety, depression, resentment, despair, rage, and any other dysfunctional feelings that roil beneath the surface of our awareness. Variations of protest—"No! Don't risk it! You can't!"—come bubbling to the surface. I believe such resistance is actually an essential and natural part of the process of manifesting. In fact, the more empowering your creative endeavor, the more bubbling up there is likely to be. The more you resist it, the more you suffer, losing connection to your own power. Sometimes this occurs before you manifest, other times right after.

For example, think of times when you have bought a new car or a house—something significant or that stretched you financially. Did you experience "buyer's remorse"? Did you feel afraid something might be wrong with it, freak out at the termite report, and then have a contraction that said, 'I knew this wasn't the right one to buy, I should've…'?

Often, expansion beyond our own comfort zone brings up fear. Even though someone else might see your purchase or achievement as good fortune and assume you should only feel happy, the truth is, when we don't address those niggling anxieties, they gnaw away at our feeling of achievement.

This is especially true for the powerful manifestation of giving birth. During labor there is a final stage before the actual pushing called *transition*. Transition is generally the shortest part of labor, lasting 15–30 minutes on average. As the labor contractions become more frequent, they last longer and for many women become the most intense part of labor. As they were delivering their first babies, two different students whom I was assisting as a labor coach each turned to me in this transition phase and whispered in a panicked voice, "I can't keep going—I just don't think I can do it." In fact, the major emotional marker for this stage of birthing is an intense desire to give up. Likewise, when something you have envisioned is on the brink of materializing, the process can be as intense as a firewalk. How you experience the emotion of that intensity is up to you. In his remarkable and straightforward book, *Thresholds of the Mind,* Bill Harris writes:

> Upheaval is part of life, and if you're on a path of growth, you'll experience more of it than if you hide from growth. When you resist upheaval as it occurs, you suffer. When you let it be okay, however, you may feel intensity, but you will not suffer over it …Many experiences in life have intensity, and this intensity can be positive, negative or neutral, depending on whether we welcome it, resist it, or are ambivalent toward it. Most people assume the quality of intensity they feel in a given situation is intrinsic to that experience, but it's actually a result of the *meaning* they place on the experience. For that reason, an intense experience, if it isn't resisted, may still be intense, but not in a negative way. [1]

Using Everything

Learn to wish that everything should come to pass exactly as it does.
— *Epictetus*

Things are going to bubble up from below the surface as you make the choice to own your power. If you accept the tenet that everything in your life not only has value, but is actually essential to the fulfillment of your potential, you'll have more capacity to trust your process and be in your power. You'll know where you are rooted and understand what has brought you to this moment, rather than having your unconscious fears or outworn beliefs dictate your reactions or throw you off-center because you haven't really addressed them.

This, then, is the essence of the Practice *Allow Alchemy*—letting there be space for any and all fear, doubt, or anxiety and then learning to transform that energy. Here, you become aware of anything that would make you resist "what is," inviting the light of Heaven to shine on the darkness below the surface, just as the sun heats up compost and transforms it into nourishment.

Denial: Garbage Stuffed in a Closed Plastic Bag

We attempt to think our way into right actions instead of act our way into right thinking.
— *Julia Cameron*

When garbage is trapped inside plastic bags, it putrefies, and its usefulness ceases. It's only when that bag splits open and allows the rotten contents to be exposed to air and earth that it can rejoin the cycle of reciprocity that is the natural order.

Likewise, when we are "in denial" and totally closed to looking at "what is," we shut down our awareness and ability to compost what needs to change in our life. Stuck in the eddy of a repeating dysfunctional pattern, we might choose to ignore whatever is troubling us, try to "rise above" it, or blame our problems on someone else. In essence, we've tied up our own "garbage" in a bag.

Let's take, for example, a woman, Alice, whose stepson, Jason, an inveterate gambler, sometimes asked her for a loan to help him cover rent and utilities, a loan which he rarely, if ever, repaid. Angered by this past behavior, Alice blamed him and his "irresponsibility" when she didn't have enough money to go away with her friends for a weekend. When Jason again asked her for money, which he said was to cover medical bills for his daughter, Alice didn't want to confront him about other times when he'd said he simply didn't have the money to repay her.

She told me she was actually grateful Jason shared his problems with her and "treated her like family," and that this time she was certain he would really pay her back as he'd vehemently promised. Although Alice lived on a small fixed income, she took out a second mortgage on her home to "help him out" once more.

I think Alice fell into the trap of "either/or" thinking, where her stepson was either "good" or "bad." This split kept her from being able to make a choice based on the whole of what she knew. If, instead, she had acknowledged the impact of his past actions, including her now-buried concern that he wouldn't ever repay her, she'd be making her choices from her true integrity. Even if she still chose to lend him some money, she could do so in a way that would have included some very specific limits.

This kind of denial, in which Alice couldn't acknowledge her resentment about not being repaid and, furthermore, had again convinced herself that "this time will be different" is, I believe, like locking her knowledge into a knotted plastic bag, away from the "earth" of her past experience and the "air and light" of the discernment of her Observer Self. When someone is unwilling to work with what is, only putrefaction can result. There is no food for growth here, only a decaying sense of self.

A friend of mine told me she bought a pumpkin for Halloween unlike one she had ever seen before. With its extremely hard surface, it reminded her of Cinderella's pumpkin carriage. So taken with it, she didn't carve it. She set it on her front porch and just left it there, marveling at how beautiful it was.

Months later, she noticed the top was caving in a little. Although the rest of the pumpkin still looked perfectly solid, she decided it was time to throw it away. When she tried to pick it up, it cracked open in a dozen places, and the insides of the pumpkin, now just liquid and seeds, gushed out over the stoop and down the sidewalk. The solid appearance on the outside had been hiding the rotting process going on inside.

Sadly, I believe this is what happens to many of us during certain times. By the time we open our eyes to the degree of destruction we've accumulated within ourselves, or within our relationships, it's too late to salvage even the parts we dearly cherished.

The Alchemical Process: Working the Soil

Garbage helps things grow! One thing rots, something else flowers or ripens because of it!
— Dr. Monza Naff

Given that this is the Earth triad, composting is, I believe, a helpful model for how to "use everything" and allow alchemy to happen at its most profound levels. The composting process is a perfect metaphor for how to work with challenging issues as they appear. I believe you can transform used-up, toxic ways of being into new discoveries and healthy choices that nourish your process of manifestation.

When I moved to my house in Oakland, I started a new garden. However, the soil was so thick with clay that after several years, I decided the main thing I wanted to grow was good dirt. I researched permaculture and spent two years covering and recovering the entire backyard with newspaper and a mix of alfalfa and straw. Although I did do some plantings directly into the alfalfa piles, my main focus was watching straw break down. In addition, I had two compost bins and a worm bed. I found growing rich loamy dirt over that period of time was a fun and easy project that took very little of my time or energy.

While some things I learned in the process were things I already knew intellectually, I took in the lessons on a deeper level as I worked to compost my yard. One was that compost happens no matter what you do.

When you create a compost pile, you have a choice of how to go about it—you can either work it or not. With "cold" compost, you simply throw clippings and food scraps into a pile, and then leave it alone to break down over time. With a "hot" compost pile, you provide the optimal conditions for the organisms to decompose faster by balancing air, moisture, and the proper ratio of dried leaves, straw, grass clippings, etc. If you choose, you can also turn the pile with a pitchfork to aerate it and distribute the moisture. The combination of all of these components causes the pile to heat up and break down old matter. In other words, with hot compost you intentionally *accelerate the process by creating an optimal environment* for an alchemical transformation to take place.

The Cold Compost Approach

The difference between cold and hot compost is determined by how much you work the pile. In the same way, your process of transformation will be affected by how you choose to work the soil of your own personal development. The speed of transformation—if you choose not to give it much energy—may be tediously slow, can even take a lifetime (or, as reincarnation would suggest, many). The problems you are facing may wear away in time, but the process will take a lot longer and may attract added problems—the gnawing rodents of worry, self-doubt, or unwanted consequences that are drawn to stagnation.

For example, Mary had a big argument with her brother Ted when she saw him over the holidays. Feeling she could no longer talk to him, she was burdened with irritation and worry for months afterwards. She told me, "I've had it! He's impossible!" Although she and Ted had shared a strong bond since childhood, she was busy, and put the matter of resolving their differences on hold until a better time. When they finally saw each other a year later, both of them felt less attached to their conflicting positions and were able to resolve their issue. In fact, the resolution came easier than either one had imagined. Ted told Mary he had been "dreading" their next encounter and was relieved. She told me they had both realized they had wasted a fair amount of time feeling anxious and distant, although, after time, their conflict had become less charged and easier to resolve.

The Hot Compost Approach

Just as you speed up the process of breaking down waste materials by intentionally creating a balance of different ingredients, to cultivate the "ground" that supports and nourishes your transformation depends on how you combine several factors. What these ingredients are and how they balance one another may well vary from one person to the next. Only you know what conditions are optimal to support you both externally—resources, people, and events—and internally—the thoughts, feelings, and attitudes that are your inner landscape.

In order to accelerate the alchemy of a hot compost pile, the primary ingredients to balance are air and light, moisture, "browns" (dead matter) and "greens" (live matter). When you think about times you have "composted" something in your life, or changed what no longer served you into something new, you could use the analogy of these ingredients to consider some primary questions:

1. Air and Light: *Where do you put your attention and awareness?*

When a compost pile gets too compacted, it cannot access light and air and thus becomes stagnant. Likewise, if you do not oxygenate or give space to whatever you are working to change, you can end up snuffing out your own light of inspiration. Letting go of denial, and cultivating the Observer, listening to your guidance, and, most important, remembering to breathe through the process are all ways to add the air and light necessary to transformation.

2. Moisture: *How do you feel about your own process?*

Feelings relate to water, especially when they are expressed through tears of joy or sorrow. They provide the moisture that accelerates the composting process. I believe it's particularly critical to cultivate compassion for yourself and others during times of change—especially when you find things breaking down in your life, where something is just not "going right." Cultivating inner kindness in the face of adversity is immensely helpful. Staying connected to your heart, loving yourself and others as you do your inner work is like adding moisture to the compost pile, providing the lubrication needed to get yourself going, align with your intention, and stay connected to joy as a fuel. Moisture and fluidity are, after all, key ingredients for providing a fertile environment for creation of any kind.

3. Browns: *What do you need to learn from the past about what no longer serves you?*

I believe it's always important to access the understanding that comes from past experience. At the same time, we should not allow the past, such as old habits and/or unresolved conflicts, determine the future. Like the browns in a compost pile, the past is essentially dead material. Too many browns slow down the transformation. People often decelerate change and keep themselves from venturing into new territory because of limiting messages they have come to believe, such as "Nothing will ever change," "My teacher told me I can't sing," or "I tried it already and it didn't work."

4. Greens: *What are you choosing now and what are you willing to do?*

Intention and the willingness to change are the other key factors that catalyze growth. These are the "greens" of the composting process, where what you have in front of you is still fresh and full of life force. You have the ability to make profound changes in your life whenever you choose, regardless of what is happening. It may take effort and stamina, but if we don't take the opportunity to transform the impact of challenges to our spirits, our minds, our very life-force, we risk being less than we're meant to be.

When you encounter difficulties, developing a willingness to use everything, to integrate all circumstances, insights and questions—no matter how challenging—is crucial. Integrity "turns over" and "heats up" your situation, essentially bringing the breath of the Heaven realm to aerate the density of your experience in the Earth realm.

"Hot" compost in your life is not boring or bland. When you live out your integrity— all of the aspects that make you *you*—your life becomes enlivened, more exciting and adventurous. In accordance with the Law of the Earth realm, alchemy occurs, and transmutes new energy out of the old, opening the circle of habit into a spiral of growth.

Invoking the Power of the Earth Realm

Here again are the four categories that work with the themes of the Earth triad. "Embodying" contains the physical exercises and Chi Kung forms to create the energetic support system for the Earth triad. "Illuminating" includes meditations and chants for the Earth realm. "Accessing" contains daily witnessing exercises. And "Deepening" explores how you can pivot circles into spirals, integrating your whole self and so allow the alchemy of changing straw into gold.

Warm-ups/Stretches

In addition to any of the warm-up exercises from previous Practice chapters, you may choose to add these stretches (or others you enjoy) specifically intended to ground you in the Earth triad.

Seated Grounding [2]

Sit on the ground with your legs stretched straight out in front of you with your feet flexed and toes pointing up. Place your palms on the floor by your buttocks. Circle your feet, first moving them away from each other, then pointing them straight ahead, then bringing your toes in toward one another, then completing the circle by coming back to the flexed position. Circle 9x. Then reverse directions and circle 9x. As you circle your feet, rock your body forward and back. Time your rocking so that as your body leans forward, you extend your ankles, pointing your toes. As you rock back, your toes come up in a flexed position.

Summoning the Spiral

Skip this exercise if you have a knee or back injury that would make it uncomfortable

Starting Position:

Sit on the ground on your right buttock, leaning on your right hand, and bend both knees back to your left so that your feet are tucked behind you. Your left hand is resting on the top of your thigh. Now pull your right leg out from under your left one and extend it forward so your knee is bent at a right angle and the outside of your calf and thigh are on the ground. Your right calf in front should be parallel to your back left thigh. Make sure that both of your legs are comfortable and do not feel strained. *If this is uncomfortable, you might want to place a pillow under your front knee.*

Movement:

1. Rotate your waist towards the left and sink your back (left) buttock down towards the floor. Let your left arm hang by your side.

2. Now begin a spiral motion up your spine by pressing your left hip up and forward. Continue the spiral motion by rotating your waist to the

right. Following the motion of the waist, rotate your chest and finally turn your head to the right looking back over your right shoulder. Let your left arm follow the movement, raising it up over your head on a high diagonal to the right until your fingertips come into your field of vision.

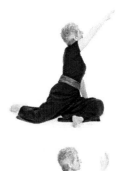

3. Ground your spiral back down in the other direction by first sinking your left buttocks back to the ground. Follow the movement of the hip by turning the waist to the left, then the chest and head, back to where you started, facing forward, allowing your arm to trail back down to your side again.

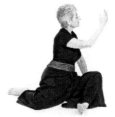

4. Do the spiral 3x, then swing your legs to the other side and repeat 3x on the other side.

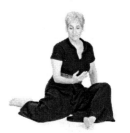

Embodying the Power of the Earth Triad with Applied Chi Kung

With the Practice of *Allow Alchemy*, you learn to compost everything that happens in your life into fuel for growth. What follows are ways to embody the themes of the Earth triad so that your cells may absorb and transform the information and energy intrinsic to it: the Heaven Law, *Circles Open into Spirals*, Human Principle, *Integrity Activates Change,* and the Earth Practice, *Allow Alchemy*. Again, you are welcome to read through the exercises, and do the ones that feel the most timely, or you can do them all in the order given.

Chi Kung to Embody the Law *Circles Open into Spirals*

Following are two Chi Kung practices to embody this Law.[3]

Transition

In the presentation of *Circles Open into Spirals,* we looked at how patterns can occur in either stagnant repetition or can be used to pivot onto a new rung of an upward spiral. This slightly longer Chi Kung form helps us to transition out of conditioned reactions and alchemize our experience into new ways of being. Developing out of the behavior embedded in the previous Practice, *Cultivate Discernment*, where you learn to distinguish what feeds you and what drains you, *Transition* creates the energetic support system in your body to make the changes you need to manifest the things you *do* want.

Given that our lives are in a constant state of change, *Transition* is a crucial tool, not only for pivoting stagnant patterns during larger life passages (such as leaving a job, ending a relationship, moving, etc.), but also for daily transitions. My Chi Kung students practice this exercise for daily or hourly changes as well (such as for therapists between clients, waitresses between shifts, or transitions from one kind of activity to another).

This form contains the six aspects to any transition: release, new growth, synthesis, expression, expansion, and contraction (rest). For this particular form, I begin each step with a question for you to consider. (Some steps have an alternate question for daily transitions). Take a moment before you do the form to consider the question for each stage of transition. Then I give you the physical and energetic instructions, as well as a short affirmation.

The Form
1. Release—*Exhale*
The first step of any transition involves some kind of letting go. Like a gardener pruning away dead wood, this movement clears your energy so that something new can emerge.

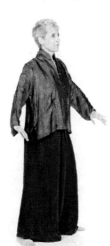

Question: What attitude or activity have you been holding onto that used to serve you but no longer contributes to your growth?

Alternate Question: What do you need to let go of right now in order to be fully present in your next activity?

Physical: Stand in a *Modified Horse Stance* with the feet hip distance apart and slightly turned out. Begin with your hands next to one another in front of the lower *tan tien*, with your palms facing down. Move your hands away from one another out past your hips.

Energetic: As you move your hands out, imagine you are letting stagnant chi release and travel down

through your legs into the earth where it can compost.
Meditation: *I release anything that no longer serves me.*

2. Draw in—*Inhale*

Pruning a plant stimulates it to produce new growth. In the same way, when you release old habits that no longer have any usefulness, you create space for new energy to enter. The new energy may be an anticipated mani-

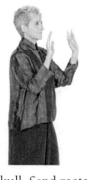

festation or one that is totally unexpected and delightful.

Question: What am I drawing in that feeds my confidence and nourishes me?

Physical: Draw the backs of your hands towards one another with your fingers pointing down. Leading with your wrists, draw your hands up the centerline of your body toward your chin.

Energetic: Imagine that the energy for this move begins at the bottoms of your feet. Draw freshly composted chi up from the earth through the soles of your feet, with a focus on your bubbling wells points (K1s). Imagine it is the chi traveling up your legs and spine that raises your arms.

Meditation: *I welcome new, nourishing energy as I move forward.*

3. Integrate—*Exhale*

The next step is to synthesize this new energy into your being. You're not trying to transform into a whole new person. Rather, you're allowing the new energy to have a transformative effect on what is happening now, so that it blends with who you already are and becomes a part of you.

Question: What do you want to remember and sustain through this time (or moment) of change?

Physical: Drop your elbows down towards the earth, turning your palms to face forward ("surrender" position).

Energetic: Imagine that someone lightly taps the top of your head, so energy travels down, aligning your spine as though your vertebrae were dangling from your skull. Send roots from the base of your spine and the bottoms of your feet into the earth. Imagine it is the release in your spine that causes you to drop your elbows with your palms facing forward.

Meditation: *I embrace my wholeness as I move forward on my path.*

4. Express (Internal Opening)—*Inhale*

This is the moment when you allow yourself to experience the transition internally. In the context of this form, the word "express" refers to an action that is inward and contemplative. Here you nourish yourself by expressing yourself for your own benefit, as you might do when you write in a journal, doodle, sing in the shower, or take the time to just listen to yourself. As you give attention and chi to your internal shift, the external wei chi is activated in the solar plexus by your inhalation.

Question: What does your inner sense tell you about your transition?

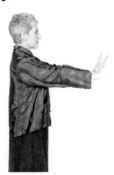

Physical: From the surrender position in the previous step, push your hands straight forward from the chest, heart level.

Energetic: Inhale as you push your palms forward. Expand your lungs (the organs in Chi Kung that represent courage) for your transition. Drawing your breath inward while pushing your hands outward is a particularly Taoist movement because it contains opposition. As you inhale, you affirm the yin embedded inside of the yang of your push. The movement of energy going in two opposite directions simultaneously becomes polarized and electric in its nature.

Meditation: *I give myself all the time and space I need to ride this change.*

5. Expand—*Exhale*

As you embody and radiate your transition, you become empowered, visible. This is a moment of allowing the alchemy of the transition to manifest and live. Your inner work has prepared the ground, so the manifestation of the transition becomes effortless.

Question: What do I want to feel and know at the completion of this change?

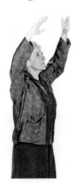

Alternate Question: What attitude do I want to have as I move into my next activity?

Physical: Raise your arms, softening your wrists so your fingertips turn toward each other, with the elbows bent slightly out, rounding your arms. When your arms are over your head, circle them out and away from each other to the sides of your body, palms out, bringing them down to just below shoulder height.

Energetic: Expand into the space around you from the internal space you have created. Imagine you fill the space

around you from the core of your spine out through the tips of your fingers.
Meditation: *I relax into the full expression of my being.*

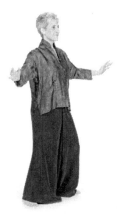

6. Contract—*Inhale*

Every expansion in Nature is followed by a contraction. Flowers open, then close. The ocean tide rushes to shore, then ebbs. Our lungs expand, then contract. The lesson here is to find ways to contract, to go back to a smaller self in a gentle self-loving way. This is the moment in the form, after your transition is completed, that you can relax, rest and replenish. It is like coming home to a candle burning in the night. Breathe in the lessons learned. Appreciate yourself and the inner work you have done during this change.

Question: As I rest and reflect, what do I hope I have learned?

Alternate Question: As I rest and reflect, what do I want in the next phase of my day?

Physical: Draw your hands back towards your lower belly. Either rest them on your lower *tan tien,* with your left hand covering right, or begin the form again from step 2.

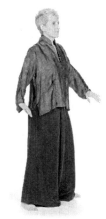

Energetic: Come back home to your center (*lower tan tien*) to rest. Take in the shift you have completed, refreshing yourself before beginning again.

Meditation: *I am mindful and present as I end this transition and begin again.*

The Pump

When your energy feels blocked, it is sometimes hard to even imagine yourself making a shift, let alone pivot to a new rung of your spiral. At those times, it is helpful to practice the *Pump,* one of Dr. Quinn's "Chi Cybernetics" that helps to circulate your blood and stimulate your energy. Sometimes all that is needed to make a change is a little aerobic stimulation. By increasing the speed when you do this form, you can jump-start the flow of your energy.

The Form

1. Draw in Energy—*Inhale.* Breathe in through your nose.

Physical: Stand in a *Modified Horse Stance*. Leading with the top of your wrists, keeping your palms down, raise your arms straight out in front of you until they are parallel to the ground, about heart level with your fingertips pointing down. At this point, as Dr. Quinn instructs, "Hold the fullness for three seconds initially, creating a suspension… (This) quiet time is of utmost importance in movement meditation sequences, because it is within this expression of intention that the chi flows in, bringing insight and illumination."[4]

Energetic: Picture chi rising from your bubbling wells points (K1s) up your legs and spine. Imagine you are drawing chi up from the earth through your roots, filling you with strength, confidence, connection to your ancestors, and the things that support you in the same way the earth herself supports the weight of your body.

2. Flush Out Stagnation—*Exhale.* Form a little "O" with your mouth as you breathe out, as though you are blowing out a candle.

Physical: Now drop the base of your wrists, so your arms swing down and back behind you, with your fingertips trailing. Go as far back as is comfortable for your shoulders.

Energetic: Imagine you are flushing out any stagnation, outdated attitudes, hooks, triggers—any thought forms or habits that keep you stuck or drained of vitality. As you swing your arms down and back, picture flushing all of that stagnation down your legs and into the earth so it can compost, transforming into neutral energy for future use.

3. Swing your Arms—*Inhale and Exhale*

Physical: As you inhale, bring your arms back up in front of you, again leading with the top of your wrists. Continue to swing your arms back and forth. Let your wrists lead and your fingers follow as though you were moving your hands though water. Keep the backs of your knees soft (slightly bent) as you swing your arms. As you build momentum, you will find you begin to bounce up and down a little in your legs. Let this happen, if it does, but don't try force it.

Guidelines: Begin the *Pump* by swinging your arms slowly, with a slight suspension in the upswing about 9x. Then let the momentum of the movement take over and increase your speed. The movement of the pump is rhythmic and powerful like the waves of the ocean, as well as relaxed and effortless, like a child enjoying a ride on a swing. Ultimately the goal is to repeat the complete arm swings 99x in a minute. Much more important than speed and tempo, however, is your internal sense of what feels right. You may want to simply do 9x and then stop, or you may want to increase speed and repetitions as you continue to practice. The main intention is to stay relaxed and focused throughout the exercise. Don't push anything and enjoy the movement! Complete the *Pump* by slowing down to your original timing for the last 5x.

Finish: When you've completed your repetitions, stand still with your hands placed over your lower *tan tien*. Breathe into your belly and let your heart slow down. Notice what you become aware of in your body, emotions and thoughts. Feel your Spirit aerated and replenished.

Chi Kung to Embody the Principle *Integrity Activates Change*

Following are two Chi Kung applications to embody this Principle.

Drawing Earth to Heaven, Heaven to Earth: The Task of the Human

T'ai   Peace

In accordance with the Principle of the Earth triad, this form places you in alignment with Heaven and Earth, where the inspiration of Heaven becomes manifest on Earth and the matter that is Earth returns to the pure energy that is Heaven.

The Form

1. Draw your energy up from the earth—*Inhale*

Physical: In a *Modified Horse Stance*, begin with your arms down by your sides. Then lift your arms with wrists relaxed. Keep them parallel as you raise them up to chest height, palms towards the ground, fingertips pointing down.

Energetic: Feel the chi rise from the soles of your feet and up your spine. Infuse yourself with a sense of grounding, confidence, the earth.

2. Surround yourself with earth energy— *Exhale*

Physical: Stretch your arms apart horizontally, extending them out to the sides of your body, shoulder height, fingers still pointing down toward the ground.

Energetic: Imagine that you are filled with and expanded by your confidence, resources, all that nourishes and sustains you.

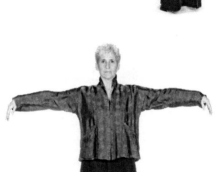

3. Integrate Yin and Yang—*Inhale*

Physical: Keep your arms where they are and in one quick movement, flick your fingers up from your wrists towards the sky. Then, bend your elbows and draw your arms over your head, with the palms turned up. Bring the tips of your fingers toward one another directly over the crown of your head, without touching.

Energetic: Draw together the different aspects of your personality into one unified whole. This is a moment of accepting and being wholly yourself.

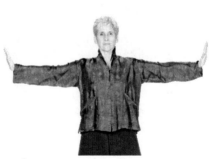

4. Now integrated, send a prayer up to the heavens—*Exhale*

Physical: With your palms still turned up

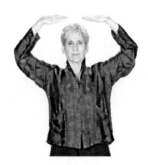

and your fingers still pointing towards one another, push your palms straight up towards the sky.
Energetic: Using your body as a conduit, move energy from the earth up to heaven.

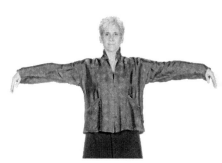

5. Receive the response that heaven rains down over you—*Inhale*
Physical: Lower your arms out to the sides, just below shoulder height, palms down (the same posture as in step 2). At the end of the move, allow your wrists to drop, so that your fingertips point down towards the earth.

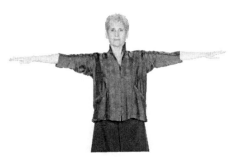

Energetic: Picture yourself showered with inspiration, visionary illumination. Open the crown of your head to receive this shower of light as it pours down over you. Breathe it in.

6. Draw the heavenly response (consciousness) around you like a cloak—*Exhale*
Physical: Draw your arms forward until they are parallel in front of your chest, palms and fingers pointing down (as in step 1).
Energetic: Let the space between your shoulder blades open. Surround yourself with the illumination and inspiration you just received from the heaven realm.

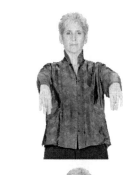

7. Draw that heavenly perspective into your body—*Inhale*
Physical: Rotate your palms, turning your fingertips in toward each other. Simultaneously, bend your elbows, drawing your hands in towards your face.

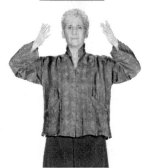

Energetic: Breathe in, drawing heavenly consciousness and guidance into your mind and body. Make it yours.

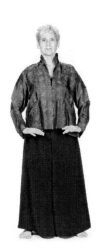

8. Ground that heavenly awareness down to earth—*Exhale*

Physical: Turning your palms down, fingertips still toward each other, press your hands down towards the ground in front of your body.

Energetic: Again using your body as a conduit, bring heaven down to earth. Infuse your whole body with heavenly consciousness as you ground yourself.

Lotus Wafting[5]

Like *Wei Chi* and *Pebble in the Lake,* which are Human triad applications, *Lotus Wafting* is a radiant, heart-centered practice. I place it here as an application for the Principle (Human/Heart aspect) of the Earth triad because it is through the Harmonious Balance (first triad Principle) and the subsequent establishment of your Boundaries (second triad Principle) that you are able to integrate all of who you are as a source of power and strength (third triad Principle). Excerpted and adapted from a longer form, the *Lotus,* this short version is, as you may remember from the previous chapter on *Integrity Activates Change,* the form that Michelle practiced after her painful encounter with the man in the park.

The Form

1. Physical: With your eyes closed, stand in a *Modified Horse Stance* with your hands placed on your lower *tan tien.*

Energetic: Take a moment to ask yourself the question: "What would I

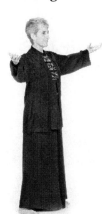

like to send out as a prayer or affirmation with this movement?" Take a moment to picture that intention radiating in your heart. You may experience it as feeling, thought, sound or image.

2. Physical: Keeping one hand cradled inside the other, rotate your palms up toward the sky. Then, keeping your hands close to your body, raise them up to heart level. Keeping your palms up, extend both arms straight out to the sides, shoulder height. Keep your hands in your peripheral vision.

Energetic: Imagine your heart opening and extending out to fill the space around you.

3. **Physical:** Rotate your waist towards the right and let your arms follow the movement. As you do, turn your head so you are looking at your right hand and the space beyond it. Simultaneously, rotate the right palm down and back and continue the backward movement. Keep your left palm turned up towards the sky. Keep your wrists relaxed. Continue to turn your waist towards the right as far as you comfortably can, while keeping your hips and pelvis facing forward so you do not twist your knees. Your arms and torso move together in one fluid movement.

Energetic: Imagine you are standing in the center of a lake with your arms floating on the surface of the water. As you turn your waist, your hands press lightly on the surface of the water, causing ripples to expand out around you.

4. **Physical:** Reverse directions. Begin to rotate your waist to the left and simultaneously rotate your right palm back to face the sky and your left palm down and back. Continue the rotation to the left, turning your head so you are looking now at your left hand and the space beyond it. Again, it is one fluid movement.

Energetic: Imagine that you are like a lotus at the center of a lake, wafting a fragrance of heart-centered chi around you, a gift that is being sent and received with love.

5. **Close:** When you have completed your repetitions, bring your hands back to your lower *tan tien*. Close your eyes and breathe into your heart.

Chi Kung to Embody the Practice
Allow Alchemy

What follows are three Chi Kung applications to embody this Practice, *Lotus Push, Water Wheel,* and *Grounding to Earth.*

The Lotus Push

Also drawn from the longer Chi Kung form called the *Lotus*, this exercise physicalizes how to be present with your feelings of resistance while at the same time opening to the detached and compassionate awareness of your Observer Self. When you do the *Lotus Push*, you practice being present with the myriad of feelings that come up during a struggle, be it external or internal. Here you are awakening a cellular consciousness of ways to resolve conflict, including how not to resist your own resistance. Through this witnessing you will find that resolution, the release of resistance and struggle, often comes to you, seemingly "out of the blue."

When the hands, a metaphor for two sides of a conflict, come to resolution at the end of the form, each recognizes it is both a part of the whole. Just as yin and yang do not exist one without the other, the two sides can move into a harmony of co-existence, finally letting go of the struggle and the suffering that resistance brings.

The Form

1. Starting Position: Stand in a *Modified Horse Stance*. With your hands at the level of your solar plexus, put the outside edge of your left palm heel (on the pinky finger side) into the hollow of your right palm. Relax the fingers on both hands so they are slightly curled. Make sure the thumb of the right hand is underneath the fingers of the left hand.

2. Physical: Use the palm heel of the left hand to push your right hand to the right until your hands are near the right side of your waist. Then, turn the fingers of the *left* hand down, shifting the angle of the right hand as though the *left* hand is starting a dive, fingers first. Use the left palm to push the right hand down until both hands descend to about hip level. Once your hands are at hip level, continue to push your left palm against the right one, moving both hands further towards the right. Allow the waist to turn to the right as well, following the direction of your hands. Rotate as far as is comfortable without straining your lower back, waist, or knees.

Focus: Here you are allowing the energy to descend towards the lower chakras so that the struggle and resistance can be played out and observed as the left hand "dominates" the right.

3. Physical: Keeping your palms pressed together, rotate your hands so that they are in the opposite position with the right hand now in place to push the left hand towards the left side of your body. Palms together, your hands pass in front of your lower *tan tien*, then all the way over toward the left hip, rotating your waist to the left as far as is comfortable.

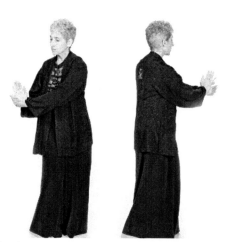

Focus: Gaze down at your hands, keeping your head and neck vertical. This embodies a posture where you can both see what is happening and experience the resistance as one hand pushes the other. As one hand pushes, the other resists, creating a state of isometric tension between your two hands. In this way, your movement symbolizes the polarized belief of win/lose, of dominance/ submission.

4. Physical: Rotate your palms again so the left hand is back in the "dominant" position. Push the left hand against the right, moving back again across the *tan tien* and turning your waist to the right once more.

Focus: As you feel resistance being played out through the pressure and resistance of one hand pushing against the other, witness it with deep compassion, remembering each voice within a conflict has its own reasoning and position.

5. Physical: When you've gone as far to the right as is comfortable, reverse the hands and change directions once more. This time, as your hands pass in front of the lower *tan tien,* continue to push your right palm against the left, but raise your arms on a diagonal to the left to about heart level. Your waist will have turned slightly so that, while you are gazing at your hands to the left of center, your hands are still in front of your heart.

6. Physical: Then turn your left hand over so that the left palm faces forward and the back of the hand now nestles into the palm of your right hand. Imagine the space between the shoulder blades, the "backbone of the heart," releases and that energy travels down your arms. Now, keeping the back of your left hand nestled in the right palm, wave your hands as though they were a sea plant being moved by a current. Begin the motion of the hands at the palm heels, lightly pressing both palms forward and releasing through the fingers.

Focus: The turning of the hands so they are nestled together symbolizes the recognition that the two sides in conflict are actually inter-dependent and that one side does not exist without the other. They are the same. As you wave your hands, you are releasing the struggle as the two sides become harmonious.

7. **Physical:** Bring both hands to rest on your lower *tan tien,* right hand covering the left hand. Stop and breathe.

Focus: This last posture is a moment of rest. It also holds the gestation of potential, of who and what we can be when we release resistance and struggle.

As you practice this exercise, really do push with one hand and resist with the other as you would in any isometric exercise. At the same time, as you exert pressure in this way, keep your neck and head loose and uninvolved so the struggle between the two hands happens at the level of your solar plexus and belly. Imagine that your head is floating effortlessly above the fray, detached from the pressure between your two hands, enhancing your connection to the Observer Self. Notice that you are not trying to stop or even ease the struggle. You're simply being present with it, so as your hands and arms work out, you practice cultivating a sense of peaceful calm—maybe even with a dash of humor.

I've included the *Lotus Push* in this chapter because it is an effective tool to address feelings of resistance. Also, with this exercise, you climb up the scale of the three *Way of Joy* Practices—from the Earth to Human to Heaven triads. By practicing the push, you *allow alchemy* to begin as you observe different inner voices strive for domination. You *cultivate discernment* when you practice identifying what each of the different elements brings to you and so recognize what to keep, what to release. Finally, in the recognition that each aspect actually is part of the whole, that in the end all aspects define and contribute one another, you *embrace wholeness (tao).*

The Water Wheel: Working Kidney Chi

The emotion that feeds the resistance to moving past old blocks is very often fear. I think this is the case because a kind of death occurs as you let go of any old forms. And death, at least for many of us in Western cultures, invokes fear. This is a common emotion whether facing a literal death of someone else, yourself, or a metaphoric death of some aspect that is no longer serving you.

In the Five Element Theory in Traditional Chinese Medicine, fear is associated with the *season* of winter, the *element* of water, and the *organ* of the Kidneys (Appendix). In his work with what he calls the Six Healing Sounds, Mantak Chia teaches that when you move energy through the kidneys, you transform fear into gentleness. This simple medical Chi Kung form circulates energy through the kidneys, nourishing them. I think it is particularly helpful when you are feeling frozen with fear, even shaken with terror.

A kindergarten teacher, who was a student of mine, began teaching some of these short Chi Kung forms in her class and nicknamed this one the *Water Wheel*. I think it is a superb image to envision as you practice this form.

The Form

Starting Position: Stand in a *Modified Horse Stance* with your feet hip distance apart and slightly turned out and your knees slightly bent. Place the *back* of your right hand on your back over your right kidney with your palm turned away from your body.

1. *Inhale:* Scoop the chi.
Physical: Shift your weight 70% to your left foot. Keeping your knees bent and the back of your right hand on your right kidney, lean forward, while simultaneously curving your elbow slightly out to the left of your body. Your arm should now be in a position to scoop up water from an imaginary pool below you. Shift your weight from your left to your right foot, continuing to lean forward. Let your left arm move with you from left to right "scooping the water."
2. *Continue the Inhale:* Continue to scoop the chi. Once you've shifted your weight 70% to your right foot, come up to a vertical position and bring your weight back to center. As you do, raise your curved arm up in

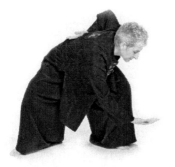

front of your body, rotating your left hand so that your palm faces forward, and continue lifting your arm until the back of your hand is in front of the center of your forehead (third eye).

3. *Exhale:* Stand still, weight centered. In your mind's eye, picture the energy you have just "scooped" traveling from your left hand down through your left arm, across your upper torso and then down your right arm into your right hand and right kidney.

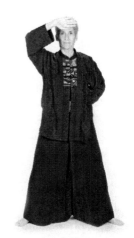

4. Do the entire exercise 3x.

5. Standing still, place your hands over your lower *tan tien* and take a moment to breathe. Feel whatever you feel, notice whatever you notice. Do you feel a difference between your two kidneys or not?

6. After a moment, do the same exercise on the other side 3x.

Close: After you have completed the exercise on both sides, stand once more with your hands covering your lower *tan tien*. Take a moment to breathe deeply into your kidneys, imagining warm energy circulating freely inside of them.

Grounding to Earth
This final exercise grounds your energy, and relaxes your Spirit.

The Form
Starting Position: Stand in a *Modified Horse Stance*. Bring your hands in front of your lower *tan tien* with your palms turned up. Place the back of your right hand on the inside of your left palm. Let the back knuckles at the base of the fingers of your right hand connect with the inside knuckles (pads) at the base of the fingers of your left hand.

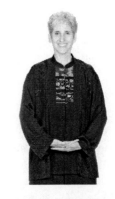

1. *Inhale*
Physical: Keeping your hands together, raise them up the centerline of your body to heart level. Keep your hands close to the body without touching it.
Focus: Imagine there is a geyser below your feet, and as the water rises, it gently pushes your hands up.

2. *Exhale*
Physical: Lower your hands back down to the level of your lower *tan tien*.
Focus: Picture the geyser slowly subsiding back down into the earth, allowing your hands to lower. Repeat 9x or more, feeling your connection to the earth. **Close:** Place your palms over your lower abdomen, keeping the left hand over the right. Focus your attention on your breath as it moves in and out.

Steep the Tea and Tapping

Complete your Chi Kung practice with *Steep the Tea* (p. 94). Then, when you get back up to stand, take a final moment to do your *Tapping* as described on page 95 to "seal in" the energy you have moved.

Illuminating the Power of the Earth Triad

For more detailed guidelines about how to enter the meditations below, see the chapters, *Embrace Wholeness* and *Cultivate Discernment*. Remember to keep your spine comfortable and aligned, whether you are sitting or lying down, and to lightly place the tip of your tongue on the roof of your mouth behind your front teeth.

Brook Meditation

This meditation calls upon imagery from the Earth to relax your body and energize your chi so that you release any blockages that keep you eddying in one place.

Preparation

Spend a few moments focusing on your breath as it moves in and out. Then bring your attention to your sitz bones, feeling them resting on the chair or cushion where you are sitting. Allow the crown of your head to lift up towards the sky, opening up space in your torso and between the bones of your spine. If you are lying down, place your focus on your tailbone and top of your head, then picture your spine lengthening along the surface you are on. Now breathe into the space between your vertebrae. As your sitz bones ground, your crown lifts, and your spine elongates, slow down your breath even more. Relax your jaw and breathe. Breathe into the space between your eyebrows.

Meditation

Picture in your mind's eye a creek or a brook. Imagine that it's a brook of bubbling chi, travelling through your body. Allow this running chi to circulate up into your ankles and knees, up your legs into your hips, lower belly and back. Let it play among the bones of your spine, circulate through your neck and shoulders, travel down your arms into your elbows, wrists and joints of your fingers. As the brook flows, let your joints relax and open. Allow the brook's water to flow into open spaces, gently washing away any held stagnation, moving through any areas in your body or mind that feel tight or stuck—incessant brain mutter, contracted muscles, feelings of fear, anxiety, or any other blockages that prevent you from experiencing the effervescence of this flowing water.

Imagine that this little giggling brook is releasing and washing anything you are holding onto that keeps you stuck or muddied, activating a balance of motion and stillness. Continue to focus on your breath as the brook of energy circulates through your body, eddying in some areas, then bursting free in a perfect balance of motion and stillness.

When you feel a tingling or sense of relaxation, slowly begin to wiggle your fingers and toes, and move your body a little, waking yourself up.

Three-Minute Refresher

Because our lives tend to be so busy, people often feel they don't have time to meditate. I wrote this meditation as a reading practice—that is, to be practiced as you read it—for those days when you need a "quick fix" to help you align Heaven, Human and Earth, but are feeling crammed. Taking only a few minutes to do, this meditation can be practiced anytime. Some people have found it useful to tape a copy of it to a place where they can remember to read it at least once during the day.

Meditation

Take a deep breath and lengthen your spine. Raise the crown of your head. Relax the space between your eyebrows, your shoulders, your jaws.

Breathe in, then out

Imagine the bones of your spine are dangling down from the crown of your head to your tailbone like a string of pearls. Relax your buttocks.

Breathe in, then out

Imagine the base of your spine, your sitz bones and the bottoms of your feet are connected to the earth, grounding you in confidence, connecting you to your biological and spiritual ancestors. Take a moment to appreciate the abundance you already have. Know there is even more to available to you.

Breathe in, then out

Open your crown to Heavenly guidance, Source, the part of you that is wise and brilliant beyond what you have yet tapped into.

Breathe in, then out

Now picture yourself as being fully free to be as big as you are. Feel the power and strength of your body and the ways in which you are agile.

Breathe in, then out

Let your arms rest on your legs with your hands turned up. Imagine that your palms and the crown of your head are catching rays from the sun, moon, stars, and other heavenly bodies. Relax your solar plexus. Release your chest and the space between your shoulder blades. Feel your feet planted and align your legs to support your arms and hands. Imagine sap rising from the earth below, giving tensile strength to your whole body.

Breathe in, then out

Open your heart. Sense yourself radiating out heart energy, then receiving heart energy.

Breathe in, then out

In the center of your wei chi (protective energy), relax completely as you give and receive.

Breathe in, then out

Appreciate the exquisite tenacity of your Spirit, the magnitude of your gifts.

Breathe In Appreciation, Breathe out Gratitude
Breathe in Trust, Breathe out Peace

Breathe in Love, Breathe out Love

With every breath, you are creating an infinite, balanced, energetic loop of reciprocity with the world around you, as you

Breathe in, then out

Earth Realm Chant

This meditation is a chant that keeps focus specifically on the Earth area of your body, from your lower belly down through your legs and feet. When we get stressed, we tend to zoom up into our minds and forget we have a body, even though it may be giving us all kinds of signals that we need to do something different, such as a tight solar plexus, clenched jaw or aching shoulders or back. You can use this chant to come back to your body, to ground and center yourself.

Sit or lie down in a comfortable position. Place your palms on your lower *tan tien*, one hand over the other. As you did with the first chanting practice in Chapter 5, *Embrace Wholeness,* relax your throat. Using the lower, deeper range of your voice, take a deep breath and tone the syllable *om*. Feel the vibration of the sound traveling into the bones of your pelvis, legs and feet. Then allow the sound to vibrate from your base up through your whole body. Repeat the sound 3–9x.

Now, keeping your eyes closed, take a moment to breathe and open your non-visual senses. Notice whatever you notice through your hearing, feeling, taste, and smell. Let these senses fling wide open, stretching beyond where they might usually go. Notice whatever thoughts may be traveling through your mind. Just observe what you perceive without getting caught in trying to evaluate what it is or create a narrative about it; rather, just witness with a sense of curiosity. Keep half of your awareness on whatever information you are tracking, and half of your awareness on your breath as it moves in and out. Stay inside of this present moment, observing the information your body brings you. Whenever you are ready, move your fingers and toes, then move your spine a little and open your eyes.

Accessing the Power of the Earth Triad in Your Daily Life

Choose one of these exercises to practice throughout this next week. Then, over the next several weeks, try another observation exercise, then another. Stay with one exercise for at least a week. Take time at the end of each day to jot down some notes about your observations.

Accessing Alchemy: Drinking It In

This exercise stems from Masaru Emoto's fascinating work with the *Hado,* "the intrinsic vibrational pattern at the atomic level"[6] of water, which has demonstrated that a word written on a water bottle can change the crystalline structure of that water. As you wake up in the morning and think about the day ahead, ask yourself "What attitude or emotion would best serve me today?" "What would move me toward a feeling of confidence or accomplishment instead of staying stuck and/or trying to avoid doubt or anxiety?" Pick a word that, even if you don't feel it at the moment, would be useful to embody, such as momentum, ease, enjoyment, compassion, courage. Write the word on a paper label and tape it to your water bottle or to a glass that you drink from throughout the day. Place the same water container by your bed at night so that you sip from it from time to time during your dreamtime if you wake up. Keep the same word on the bottle for a week, or change it when you want to. You will, in essence, be drinking water that has the "structure" of the attitude or emotion you want to internalize. Imagine the potential impact, given that such a large percentage of your body is made up of water.

Accessing the Witness—Invitation to the Unconscious

The focus here is to continue the daily practice of checking in during the day with your Observer Self. The goal is to strengthen the work you've done with the two previous "Accessing the Witness" exercises. First, as you did in this exercise in *Embrace Wholeness*, take a moment when you are feeling stressed, resistant or overly amped-up to check in with your Observer Self and watch how you are filtering information: through images, sounds, feelings, or inner dialogue. What you are saying to yourself?

Second, as you did with this exercise in *Cultivate Discernment*, notice if you are focusing on things that you don't want; if so, ask yourself what you *do* want.

Third, here, in *Allow Alchemy*, hold the focus on what you do want for a few moments, then send a message to your unconscious mind, asking it to surprise you with solutions that will help you make the shift. With this practice, you don't spin your wheels in problem-solving, but rather surrender to an inner wisdom. Then notice through the day what answers or directions come to you.

Accessing Nourishment

During one meal, take some time to focus only on your eating. This exercise is best done if you are alone unless your companion(s) would like to participate as well. Notice not *what* you eat, but *how* you eat. Avoid diversions such as reading, watching TV, or working at your computer. Your challenge here is simply to nourish your body and senses with the activity of eating. Take a moment to reflect on the source of your food. How did it come to be on your plate? As you chew and swallow, reflect, for example, on the seed or animal, the farmer, the drivers, the store. Let your imagination trace your food back to its source(s).

Become aware of whether you are chewing fast or slowly, if your mind is racing or calm, if you are breathing between bites. Now chew slowly, taking time to absorb the "lineage" of this nourishment. One of my early T'ai Chi teachers recommended chewing each bite 29 times, and I have seen variations on this kind of mindful eating in many Buddhist and Taoist practices. When you are finished with your meal, take a moment to place your palms on your belly, lean back in your chair, and focus on your digestive tract before going to your next activity.

Accessing Grounding

Take a moment during the day to lie down on the ground in a safe place (outside, if at all possible). Close your eyes and focus on your breath. Imagine you are lying down on the palm of the hand of the earth. Relax your mind and use the time to simply *Be*.

Deepening the Power of the Earth Triad: Journal Exercises

The first three exercises are rapid writes, followed by longer journal exercises. Once again I have suggested times for the rapid writes. I've found over many years of teaching that, while the idea of writing on one prompt for 2-3 minutes can initially sound like a long time, in practice my students have often experienced that one minute is not long enough. In addition, continuing to free-write after you think you are "done" or get blocked can take you to deeper insights which may surprise you.

Remember that the goal is to strike a balance that allows you to explore suggested themes more deeply while keeping the process short enough that you do not end up sabotaging yourself and not doing the exercise because you don't have time or because you feel overwhelmed. This journaling should be as easeful as possible.

Defining Your Empowerment

Recommended Time: 2-3 minutes for each part.
I can feel my power most when I . . .
The signs that let me know I am in my power are . . .
The qualities that I believe make me feel most powerful are . . .

Moving Ahead

Recommended Time: 3 minutes for each part
What I most want to create/have in my life is...
My next step to manifest that is...

What could stop me is…
I can keep that from stopping me by…

Rapid Write Exercise for Transitions

This next journal exercise is an enhancement of the Chi Kung form *Transition*, which you learned earlier in this chapter. It opens up a little more time and space for exploring the question you already considered in the practice form, so it is especially useful for major life transitions. If you'd like to practice the form after completing the writing exercise, put any feelings and thoughts generated by your journaling on the back burner so you can simply allow the energy you have generated by writing to flow through you without getting stuck in your head.

I've included a reminder for each of the six stages of *Transition*, followed by a writing prompt. This is an affirmation to set your intention into motion, so even if you don't believe you've completed the transition you are working on, write it as if you have.

Recommended Time: 1 minute for each part.

1. *What am I letting go of?* What are the qualities you feel in your body, heart, mind or spirit that seem stagnant, patterns that no longer contribute to your growth?
   Write: *I am releasing …*

2. *What do I need to nourish me?* The energy you've released into the earth composts and transforms into energy that will nourish and support your growth. The energy could be the courage to take a risk or to stand your ground in a conflict. Physically, the energy might feel effervescent like champagne rising up your legs. Notice the emotions you feel.
   Write: *I am drawing in . . .*

3. *What do I want to keep from my past experience?* As new energy comes in, you integrate new information with what you already know. In this way, you acknowledge and carry forward life lessons that are still useful at the same time you allow new changes to be synthesized.
   Write: *Trusting this transition, I know from my experience that . . .*

4. *How is this transition changing me?* This is the time when the alchemical shift happens as you open internally to allow space to be nourished.
   Write: *Inside, I know that this change means …*

5. *How has my energy changed in the external world?* This is the moment of empowerment. Like Picasso effortlessly painting in his garden

after days of internal work, this is when the product of your inner work can flow through you as your transition becomes manifest. Write: *The energy I am emitting now is …*

6. *How do I want to reflect on this change I'm making?* After completion comes rest. Here is the time to regroup, relax and appreciate the work you have done to stay mindful during a time of big change. Write: *As I relax, I can now appreciate …*

Conversation Among the Selves

Many disparate voices live in the underground of the unconsciousness. Some voices we like and some we don't, some are immature (even if they have been there forever!) while others are seasoned and wise.

Inspired by the innovative work with "Voice Dialogue," the powerful and innovative tool developed by pioneer psychologists, Drs. Hal and Sidra Stone, this writing exercise offers a way to allow some of those different internal "voices" to speak.[7] By listening to these voices, we can reclaim all of who we are and begin the process of integration so intrinsic to the Earth triad. This exercise is especially useful when you find yourself in a situation where you are feeling blocked or conflicted.

The Conversation

Begin by taking a deep breath. Then take a little time to do a free write about whatever issue is concerning you. Lay the situation out—set the stage, so to speak—for your conversation. In fact, you might think of your psyche as a play with many different characters (some voice dialogue coaches suggest thinking of your whole Self as a Company or Organization and the different aspects as employees).

Give a name to each character such as the "Healthy Self," the "Creative Self," the "Wise One," the "Inner Critic," or the "Doubter." As you work with this paradigm, you will find there are many voices that can appear in different contexts. Some clients and students, finding certain aspects had male or female qualities, have given their voices "real" names, such as Abe for the Doubter, Katrina for the "Healthy Self" or Pearl for the "Wise/Enlightened One."

Invite the various sub-personalities to a negotiating table. Include one you might call the "Mediator" or the "Detached, Compassionate One." Write down what these respective aspects say, creating a dialogue. The role of the "Mediator" is to ask questions, listen carefully, and assume that no matter how harsh, every aspect has something of value to offer to the whole system (you). It is a good idea to include some ground rules, such as "speak your truth with respect," so you do not give free rein to any train of thought that might hurt or block the process.

For example, take this dialogue from Clara, who wanted to follow a long-held dream to try some oil painting, yet felt stuck. Her "Doubter" kept saying, "Cut it out, you're such an idiot. You're always doing stuff that isn't practical. It's never gonna work, you'd be a lousy artist." Here it was important for the mediator to slow things down. The Mediator begins:

> "I know you, Doubter, are concerned that this idea is too risky. Are you worried that something will happen to Clara if she goes ahead with this plan?"
>
> "Yeah, the last time she went off and tried something and failed, she ended up feeing miserable and not doing anything for days. I'm sick of it!"
>
> "So are you trying to protect Clara from feeling bad about herself?"
>
> "I guess so, yes."
>
> "So while Clara would like your help in discerning what pitfalls may lie ahead when she ventures into new territory, if you speak to her in a harsh tone, she is more likely to resist and fight back. If you speak to her with respect, she would be better able to hear your specific concerns."

As you experiment with this process, stay open to surprising voices that may come up. Write what they have to say, and remember to ask questions about the deeper message they are trying to convey. Your Mediator aspect should continue to hold a boundary so you don't end up spiraling down in to self-blame or angst.

Transforming Worry: A Time Travel

Have you ever heard the saying, "Worry is praying for what you do not want"? Because worry keeps our attention directed towards what is stagnant or blocked, I believe anxiety about things that "might happen" is one of the greatest depleters of chi. The following writing exercise is a useful tool to address resistance that appears as anxiety about what might (or might not) happen, or fear of the unknown.

I was originally introduced to this exercise, written by Dr. Quinn, during a year-long intensive called the Five Levels. I have used it countless times in my own life as well as with students. It can be applied to many situations, including when you are about to see someone who intimidates you or with whom you're in conflict, or when you are about to face some other challenge.

Take as much time as you need. Some situations will feel more complex and will need more time than others.

On a piece of paper or in your journal, write the following prompt:

The Prompt

I just completed (or spoke with)_____. It went better that I could have possibly imagined. I was completely grounded and centered as well as flexible and compassionate. When s/he/it_____, I _____ . . .

The Directions

Blank No. 1: After the first sentence, "I just completed_____," fill in the blank with the name of the upcoming task or encounter that you are worrying about. Be sure to keep it in the past tense. For example, instead of writing *"I am about to have a meeting with my boss,"* you'd write *"I just met with my boss,* or *"I just said goodbye to my in-laws who were here for the weekend,"* or *"I just completed my taxes,"* or *"I just had a conversation with Michael,"* and so on.

Blank No. 2: In the next blank, insert the challenge you are anticipating that worries you. For example, *"When he told me he wasn't happy with the work I had done on the Bellweather project,"* *"When my mother-in-law criticized me,"* *"When I got overwhelmed trying to gather information to fill out the forms,"* and so on. This is the place to let yourself imagine everything "bad" that you're worried might happen, anything that could de-rail you or create consequences you don't want.

Blank No. 3: In the final space, "I_____," imagine yourself looking back at your responses and behaviors after having succeeded beyond your wildest expectations. Imagine acknowledging what you were able to accomplish in the face of every stressor you were worried about. For example, *"I took a deep breath and told her that her comments hurt my feelings because her respect it means a lot to me."* Or, *"I felt confident as I asked my boss what he didn't like about my work on the Bellweather project and we had a great discussion about where to go from here."* You may have more than one response you want to name. For example, *"I asked my boss if he'd like to see the research I did as the basis for how I approached the project."*

You can also repeat both the "when s/he/it/they _____," followed by the "I _____" phrases as many times as you like until you picture yourself having addressed every single aspect that concerns you.

I think one of the reasons this exercise is so effective, even prophetic, is that it breaks down the time continuum, allowing your consciousness to travel into a future where you not only feel relieved of the pressure you were experiencing, but excited about the lessons you learned from your transformative work. It gives you a new blueprint of how to get from here to there.

Conclusion: Putting it All Together

Out of the *awareness* of the Heaven realm where you *Embrace Wholeness* and the *intention* of the Human realm where you *Cultivate Discernment,* you arrive at the transformational opportunities in the Earth realm's *Allow Alchemy.* Here, you ground your power, owning your ability to live in integrity, enhancing your capacity to break through the eddy of repetitive circles and move up to a new ring in the spiral.

While we can use every Law, Principle, and Practice in the book to transform our lives, the Earth aspect of the Earth triad is the ultimate grounding, where we compost "everything" to manifest new growth. Therefore, the Earth Practice offers us the opportunity to take quantum leaps in how we work with all the other Laws, Principles and Practices. Here you can take stock of any circumstance in your life and access the appropriate tool to strengthen the energetic support system for your body, mind and spirit. This is the seed of empowerment.

To this end, I asked my students to describe various challenges they were facing that brought up feelings for which they would like a *Way of Joy* "prescription." Without going into any details of their stories, I would like to offer a distillation of the common themes in their requests and my suggestions for which Chi Kung exercises to use. You may want to use this list as a guide for times when you encounter these feelings.

I invite you, as you consider the themes of the Laws, Principles, and Practices, to think about your own life and how you would apply these or any other exercises to *Allow Alchemy,* to empower your whole being.

Suggested Remedies for Interruptions to Your Joy

In situations where I have suggested one or more exercises to choose from (or you may decide to do them all), the page numbers are listed after *each* exercise. In other situations, where I have recommended a series of exercises to be performed in sequence, the page numbers are listed *at the end of the line.*

Anger: *Space Shake* (p. 154), *Solar Plexus Bowl* (p. 164), *Wei Chi* (p. 157)

Anxiety/Worry: *Solar Plexus Bowl* (p. 164), *Eye of the Storm* (p. 88)

Arrogance/Superiority: *Pump* (p. 240), *Lotus Balance* (p. 91), *Grounding* (p. 251)

Betrayal: *Pump* (p. 240), *Earth to Heaven* (p. 242), *Shower* (p. 93)

Change/Life Transitions: *Transition* (p. 236), *Grounding* (p. 251)
   Lotus Waft (p. 245)

Depression: *Space Shake*, *Pump*, then *Shower* (p. 154, p. 240, p. 93)

Despair: *Water Wheel* (p. 249), *Shower* (p. 93), *As Above, So Below* (p. 154)

Disempowered: *Lotus Push* then *Wei Chi* (p. 247, p. 157)

Exhaustion: *Pump* (p. 240) *Water Wheel* (p. 249)

Fearful: *Water Wheel* (p. 249), *Alignment* exercise, (Part 1 and 2) (p. 152, p. 168)

Grief: *Pump* (p. 240), *As Above, So Below* (p. 154) *Pebble in the Lake* (p. 156)

Hatred: *Lotus Push* (p. 246), *Fountain* (p. 159)

Irresolvable Conflict: *Grounding, Eye of the Storm, Fountain* (p. 251, p. 88, p. 159)

Isolation/Alienation: *Earth to Heaven* (p. 242) *Fountain* (p. 159)
   Lotus Push (p. 246)

Jittery/Stage Fright: *Grounding*, then *Wei Chi* (p.251, p. 157)

Longing/Yearning: *As Above, So Below* (p. 154), *Lotus Push* (p. 246),
   Lotus Balance (p. 91)

Low Self-Esteem: *Pump*, then *Shower*, followed by *Wei Chi* (p. 241, p. 93, p. 157)

Making a Decision/Feeling Split: *Eye of the Storm, Lotus Balance, Shower*
   (p. 88, p. 91, p. 93)

Overwhelm: *Grounding* (p. 251), *Eye of the Storm* (p. 88), *Steep Tea* (p. 94)

Reactive Instead of Responsive: *Space Shake* (p. 154), *Transition* (p. 236)
   As Above, So Below (p. 154)

Remorse: *Pebble in the Lake* (p. 156), *Lotus Wafting* (p. 245) *Water Wheel* (p. 249)

Resistant: *Lotus Push* (p. 246) *Water Wheel* (p. 249) *Transition* (p.236)

Sending Love/Support: *Pebble in the Lake* (p. 156), *Lotus Wafting* (p. 245)

Self-Empowerment: *Fountain*, then *Wei Chi*, then *Pebble in the Lake* (p. 159,
   p. 157, p. 156)

Shame: *Grounding, Shower, Earth to Heaven* (p. 251, p. 93, p. 242)

Stuck: *Pump* (p. 240), *As Above, So Below* (p. 154) *Shower* (p. 93)

Victimized: *Wei Chi*, followed by *Shower* (p. 157, p. 93)

As we come to the end of our journey through the three realms, may we always remember to *Allow Alchemy* by aerating with the breath of Heaven the composting Earth of our manifest lives. Just as yin and yang, Earth and Heaven, exist one inside the other, may we remember as we embody our Spirits, that our Spirits also enfold our bodies. Thus we complete one cycle moving from Heaven to Earth, to end and begin again.

CHAPTER 12
Conclusion
Bringing Joy Home

The *Way of Joy* is a journey that leads you home to your Self, where you feel totally alive and fully present in the Now, able to embrace all that life brings. The material in this book is intended as a map for traveling through the realms of consciousness, intention, and empowerment that are intrinsic to the Taoist concepts of Heaven, Human, and Earth. I'd like to provide a synopsis of that "map" so that you'll have it available for a quick review whenever you need it.

Synopsis

It may be helpful to remember that all Laws are Heaven, all Principles are Human, and all Practices are Earth. What follows is a quick summary of these three elements.

Heaven: Home of Consciousness

The Observer is the primary presence in all three of the Laws in each of the triads. Born out of the first Law in the Heaven triad, *Within Motion, Stillness; Within Stillness, Motion,* it is within the breadth and breath of this paradox of stillness and motion that we first access the Universal Consciousness of the Observer. As human beings, when we experience a level of consciousness beyond what we normally possess, it translates as insight, a moment of illumination.

Within the second Law, in the Human triad, *Chi Moves in the Space Between,* the Observer is the presence that perceives the pregnancy of the void from which all things emerge and to which they return, opening up possibilities we have heretofore not imagined. Here we are able to conceptualize how to turn inspiration into workable concepts that can be applied in our own lives.

Within the third Law, in the Earth triad, *Circles Open into Spirals,* the Observer holds a context within which we develop clarity about our own patterns. Here we gain understanding of how to pivot out of repeating dysfunctional habits and grow into a new awareness of how to create the life we want.

Human: Home of Intention

The unifying thread of the Principles is crafting intention out of inspiration for our own unique self-expression. Here we conceptualize how to implement those moments of inspired consciousness and make them work in the world of human relationships.

The first Principle in the Heaven triad, *Balance Brings Harmony*, calls us to the vital task of keeping perspective in times of both contraction and expansion. Transitioning easefully between yin and yang, we create a stable relationship between Higher Self and Ego, translating inspiration into fulfilled and creative expression.

The second Principle in the Human triad, *Boundaries Dissolve Barriers,* articulates the means by which we define ourselves from the inside out, give shape to our self-expression, and make truly intimate connections with others.

The third Principle in the Earth triad, *Integrity Activates Change,* calls on us to access our full creative potential by lifting the veil of denial and accepting all aspects of who we are and what we do. Embedded in this Principle is the intention to accept "what is" without moving into victim mentality. We can then direct our actions to manifest a reality that is an expression of the whole Self.

Earth: Home of Action

The title of each Practice is actually a directive telling us what we can *do* to ground ourselves. The first Practice, *Embrace Wholeness,* which grounds the Heaven triad, is the embodiment of living consciously with the presence of the Observer. This is the action we take to prevent falling into the trap of polarities and to be fully present with all-that-is.

Within the second Practice, in the Human triad, *Cultivate Discernment,* we ground our ability to make distinctions between what feeds us and what drains us, what blocks our flow of chi and what sustains or enhances it. Here we make choices that come from the heart and are self-sustaining. In so doing we walk the path of individuation and self-definition that embodies our life purpose.

With the third practice, in the Earth triad, *Allow Alchemy,* we let everything that happens be composted into a source of energy that fuels and strengthens us. This includes resistance in all its forms—fear, inertia, despair, denial—the common companions on the road to empowerment. Working with all aspects of ourselves is essential to trusting the inherent alchemy of our process, owning our power and fulfilling our potential.

Summary Chart

Heaven Realm: *Consciousness - Inspiration*

Law	*Heaven Aspect*	**Within Motion, Stillness; Within Stillness, Motion** Consciousness of breath, Observer Self
Principle	*Human Aspect*	**Balance Brings Harmony** Transitions between yin and yang, expansion and contraction, ego and higher self
Practice	*Earth Aspect*	**Embrace Wholeness** Integrating polarities into unified experience

Human Realm: *Conceptualization - Intention*

Law	*Heaven Aspect*	**Chi Moves in the Space Between** Awareness of energy, infinite potential
Principle	*Human Aspect*	**Boundaries Dissolve Barriers** Creating boundaries, essential for self-definition, intimate connection and personal expression
Practice	*Earth Aspect*	**Cultivate Discernment** Making choices, distinguishing between what drains us and what feeds us, what blocks energy flow and what allows it to move freely

Earth Realm: *Manifestation - Action*

Law	*Heaven Aspect*	**Circles Open into Spirals** Insight needed to move out of closed circles of stagnation into spirals of expansion and growth
Principle	*Human Aspect*	**Integrity Activates Change** Integrating understanding of all facets of our experience as a framework for transformation
Practice	*Earth Aspect*	**Allow Alchemy** Utilizing all experiences as the compost to nurture and sustain fulfillment

While I have organized the Laws, Principles, and Practices into triads, the information contained within these concepts is ultimately interrelated and malleable. How you move among the triads is entirely up to you. For example, the Law of the Earth triad, *Circles Open into Spirals*, might offer needed insight as you work with the Practice of the Heaven triad, *Embrace Wholeness*. Or, an Earth realm aspect, such as the Practice of the Human triad, *Cultivate Discernment,* can bring you new understanding of how to express the Principle of the Heaven triad, *Balance Brings Harmony*, and so on.

My goal in structuring the information in the *Way of Joy* as I have is to create clearly defined and accessible guidelines for living a life enhanced by the exquisite and infinite presence of your own life force. As you move forward in your exploration, I encourage you to experiment with any of these ideas and use them in ways that best serve you as you bring forth your unique gift to our beloved planet.

By way of personal summary, I want to share another story about my relationship with my father—to demonstrate the effectiveness of this process when we work over time to achieve personal empowerment within the context of difficult long-term relationships. Such diligent effort can result not only in our own growth, but also have the added benefit of transforming the relationship and prompting spontaneous shifts in the other person's consciousness.

A Time of Reckoning

O! Listen to a jubilant song,
The joy of our spirit is uncaged.
—Walt Whitman, as adapted by Norman Dello Joio[1]

The scent of rain wafts through the room as the branches of the pines outside the window shudder in the summer thunderstorm. I sit next to my dying father's bed as he finally sleeps. I flash back to a memory of when I was a little girl and promised him I would be there for him when he died. I feel wonder and gratitude that, after decades of repeating cycles of conflict and rejection between us, I have arrived at this point, spiraled, if you will, to this moment. My father wakes up and our eyes lock. I place my hand over his heart and nod slightly. He smiles tenderly and drifts off again.

The man dying here is so different from the one I have known as a child, a teen, a young adult, and in these last ten years of slow reconciliation. My father was remote, so involved in his work as a composer that he had little or no patience for either my brothers or me. In fact, after we were grown, he would frequently comment, "I never wanted children—I just wanted to give your mother something to do."

On the other hand, I have memories I still treasure from when I was very little, such as the one I describe in the Prologue—dancing as he played music for dinner guests or listening to musical passages he'd just written when he'd invite me into his study.

I think the primary connection I felt with him was through the arts, his music in particular. Our whole family lived in an environment informed and surrounded by the music and art scene. As an adult, I look back and remember that pervasive presence of music absorbed into my very cells as a tiny child. I thrived in the vibrant musical energy that permeated our home. I didn't have a measure of how loved other children felt by their fathers or whether music was an important part of their lives. As a child, I only knew that this was my life.

I've mentioned how, from the time I was young I loved to dance, act, direct, and perform. In my heart, I knew myself to be an artist. My father always made clear to me, however, that, as a girl, I could never *really* be an artist. My primary function was to lend him an ear and be a supportive but silent presence. In fact, he got extremely irritated whenever I asserted my own artistic temperament and when, as an adult, I pursued a career in theater.

My father dismissed my desire and talents as mere idle fantasies, usually sarcastically and angrily. Gone was the sweetness of the playing together with music and dance when I was five. By the time I was a teenager, our connection had eroded and I was on my own, rebelling against his rejection and at the same time desperately wishing for his approval. Still, I always felt his tremendous power and the strength of his will imposed on me.

I determined never to be like him, and as an adult, maintaining humility was a driving force for me. Eventually, as I've said, I realized my humility was co-mingled with low self-esteem, much of which was prompted by my father's criticism. For many years, despite my own talents and successes, I was in some denial about the ways I kept my "light under a bushel," fearing that being "visible" would be tantamount to arrogance.

During the first decade of our estrangement, I struggled between resisting the power my father's rejection had over me, and hoping for reconciliation and approval. This resistance and stymied hope continued to hurt, despite my growth in other areas. We had a brief, tentative reconciliation that shattered when he realized I had entered a relationship with a woman. My internal struggle continued. While it faded somewhat over the second decade of our estrangement, I was still stuck in my own eddy.

Inertia in one area always affects other areas. To varying degrees, my issues with my father impacted my ability to consistently follow the Laws, Principles, and Practices of the *Way of Joy*. For instance, as I mentioned previously, it was hard to move effectively from expansion to contraction. While in a contracted state, I was very self-critical, mirroring my father's voice.

One significant unresolved relationship can profoundly affect our lives. At the same time, any of us can—and I did—continue to expand consciousness, maintain our intention to create holistic change, and see those changes manifest.

When I finally wrote to my father, applying the Principle of *Boundaries Dissolve Barriers*, I did, ultimately, break free from a crucial stagnant cycle and no longer felt so intimidated by him. Owning my own power, being willing to be more fully seen, I began to spiral outward.

For more than ten years, during a process of gradual reconciliation, I saw him regularly. I worked to hold my own with him, despite his continued criticism of me, his refusal to hear much, if anything, about my life—and gradually experienced subtle shifts in the energy between us. However, I still felt in some ways inadequate in the face of his disparagement and, in the process, moved in and out of my own victim mind-set.

On my next-to-last visit to his home in East Hampton, my father's wife, Barbara, left for California on a much-needed vacation. My father had slept through most of the afternoon while I made a *ziti al forno* (a baked pasta dish). In the early evening, he wheeled out of his bedroom to sit at the head of the dining room table. I brought out dinner and we sat down to eat. Eating pasta was a silent business for my father, except for a few grunts of "s'good, Vic." After he pushed away his plate, he leaned back, looked at me and proclaimed, "You know you haven't done anything with your life, Victoria. Your life is a failure."

This pronouncement didn't surprise me, as it had been a recurring theme during my past visits. But this time felt different. Whereas in the past I often felt hurt, angry or resigned, this time I felt a light amusement as I thought, "Oops, here he goes again." A bubble of delighted laughter rose from deep in my belly to tickle my heart while simultaneously I felt something like a breeze fluttering my hair. I had decided to hop on this old merry-go-round, just relax and have fun.

I smiled. "What is it, Dad," I asked curiously, "that's made you come to the conclusion that my life's a failure?" He leaned back in his chair and began to pontificate, reciting a litany of things I had done that departed from the ways he believed they should be done. When he stopped talking, I thought about what he said for a moment. Then I answered, "You know it's funny, Papa, but when I look at the various paths I've taken in my life, I realize they've all contributed to who I am now, and the work I do is actually a synthesis of much of it.

"It's true I've gone my own way and followed my own counsel. But you know, I think I got that from you. I listened recently to a taped interview you gave a couple of years ago. When you were asked whether you listened to a lot of other band music as you began to write music for bands. You practically shouted, 'NO!' It made me laugh because I so recognized that need to do things your own way. And I think that's part of your legacy to me."

"Huh," he mumbled, a little secret smile playing around the corners of his mouth as he considered what I said.

The next day, while we were playing backgammon, he blurted out, "You know your brother doesn't approve of your lifestyle and I don't either!"

"Do you mean because I'm a lesbian?" I asked.

"YES! What is it with you? How'd it happen?"

"Are you saying you want to talk about it?" Astounded, I remembered several years earlier, when I had asked him if he wanted to know anything about my life in California, my partner, or what we were doing together. He had proclaimed loudly, "No, Never. I wish she'd disappear off the face of the earth!" So in subsequent years, the topic of my "lifestyle" had been taboo.

When he said yes, he did want to talk, I told him what it had been like for me to have these feelings that I couldn't understand and was so afraid of when I was growing up, what it'd been like to grow up queer with an Italian patriarch as a father. I described how hard I tried to be with men, to become heterosexual, at the same time feeling, when I was with them, like I was fighting my own nature, doing something that felt unnatural, that some fundamental connection was missing.

My father listened carefully. "I never knew, Victoria," he said, "I never knew. Why didn't I know?"

"Because I did everything I could to hide it from you, Dad. I was so afraid that you'd reject me. And then when you did . . ."

"But you don't understand," he interrupted. "For me, as your father, it's a failure. It means that I *failed* you." So began a conversation that lasted for several hours about my feelings and his. I was finally able to tell him about the joy I found with the love of my life, and how lucky I thought we both were, knowing he had also found a soul mate in Barbara. He told me about a gay friend he knew at Julliard when he was young, about his confusion and sorrow when that young man killed himself. Then, he said, "You know, it's fine for us to say we love one another, but we needed to have this talk. I gotta say I don't understand any of it, but I can see this is the direction it's going. Gay marriage …It's gonna happen. And for me," he paused and thought for a minute, "well, I've always loved petting a cat. But I wouldn't want to pet a mouse. No, I could never pet a mouse. But I like petting a cat. I don't know what it is, but a mouse—it just seems so unnatural. But I don't know *why*. What's wrong with a mouse? I don't know what it is with me. I don't understand."

I was flabbergasted as I listened to him expound on this metaphor. I saw he had come to a new understanding, a shift in his consciousness. Although he ended by asserting, "But I still don't like it, I still don't approve," his voice sounded less harsh. In some ways, I thought he might be afraid that giving his approval would somehow close any loophole of hope that I was mistaken in my sexual identity. I smiled, loving him for this exploration and said, "I know, Dad. And still, I'm so glad, too, we finally had this talk."

Over that visit, we had several increasingly frank and previously avoided conversations about everything from my being a lesbian to my work. My study of *Powerful Non-Defensive Communication*™, what I consider to be the language of *wei chi*, flowed through me as I answered him, talked, laughed, acknowledged my limitations and claimed my strengths, comfortable and open inside of my own boundaries. The remaining barriers between us dissolved, and his irritation was replaced by curiosity as he asked questions and demanded answers. I realized to my delight I was practicing allowing alchemy. My old attitudes of rebellion/submission had fallen away, and I felt utterly free to speak my truth without once defending myself.

By the end of my visit, he urged me, "Do what you have to do, Vic. Follow your heart and don't let anyone stop you." Because this visit had felt like an exquisite and transformative closure, when my brother Justin called several months later to say my father was dying, I—caught in the middle of other commitments—was not certain I wanted or needed to go. And yet …as I sought inner stillness and opened the *space* for my discernment, my decision became clear.

My Father's Death

Ever since I arrived here five days ago, my father has spent time in and out of lucidity. On the first day, when Justin and I walk into his bedroom, my father looks at us incredulously. "*You*, you're here. I thought you were dead!"

I respond, "No, Dad, we're not dead."

My father's wife, Barbara, laughs and says, "No, Norman, They're alive and kicking. Aren't you glad to see them? You've been asking for them."

My father looks confused. "But how could that be? I thought ...I don't understand. It seemed so ...Where are we? Am *I* dead? I must be dead."

"No, Dad, you're not dead either," I take his hand.

He stares at me urgently, "But it was so real. I saw ...I knew ...I must've ...I've been in another world. I thought someone was trying to keep you from me. Are you really here? It's crazy, but I was so sure! Everything that happened felt so real. I could write a book about this. Or a symphony. It could be a terrifying symphony. And I could see. I have done such terrible things in my life. Such terrible things. I've been a monster. I know it now."

"Don't be silly, darling," Barbara says, as Justin pats his shoulder trying to comfort him.

Dad bellows, "WHAT?"

"Don't be silly, dear," Barbara repeats. "You're not a monster."

"Don't say that, NO! I AM a monster!"

Softly, I say, "Wait, he needs to say this. He just needs to get it out." And to my father, "Papa, what is it that makes you say you've been a monster?"

"I see myself that way. I can see it all. I know now what I have done."

"What do you believe you have done, Dad?" I ask.

My father groans, "I've been such a selfish man, so selfish and arrogant. I've done terrible things to the people I love." In the awe-filled silence that follows, space opens for his chi to move as floodgates of tears release. Sobbing, my father pulls in my brother's head and my head close to his chest, crying out his anguish," The guilt, oh the guilt!"

My father had clearly had an insight—perhaps just moments before we walked into the room—an enhanced consciousness about his treatment of those he loves. Barbara and Justin tried to reassure him, as people commonly do. Had they succeeded, although intending love and protection, they would have inadvertently blocked him from speaking his truth. When asked to say more, he was able to take his insight, transform it into an intention to speak the truth, and then through his tears manifest it finally, at ninety-five, by truly holding his children with love.

The next day, after Justin has said his final goodbye and returned home, my father looks at me, "Are you leaving too?"

"No, Dad," I reassure him, "I'm here to stay with you until the end."

"What's happening to me, Vic?" he asks. "What's my state? Tell me what's going on!"

"You are dying, Papa. Your body is slowly shutting down and letting go."

"Letting go of what?" he demands, incredulously.

"Of this body, your body. It's slowing down. But it's OK. You're doing just what you need to do. It'll be easier if you can relax."

"Relax?" he asks, baffled.

"Yes," I smile.

"Isn't there anything anyone can do?"

"No, Papa. I am so sorry." Tears spring to my eyes. "If there was anything else any of us could do, we would. It's just your time."

"Jesus!" he growls, "But how long? How long?"

I reply softly, "No one can say when—it takes as long as it takes. There's no way to predict, no way to know. This process is a mystery. And it is hard work."

"You know that? You understand? You're so right. How did you know? Boy, is it ever! It is …it's so hard."

Stroking his forehead, I murmur through tears, "Yes, I think it may be one of the hardest things we ever do."

My father's eyes widen. "There is a woman behind you as you are speaking. She is sitting there as bright as day, listening to everything you say."

"What does she look like?" I am intensely curious.

"I'm seeing ghosts. What's the hell's going on? Am I nuts?"

"No," I comfort him, remembering being with my uncle as he died just three years ago. "You're not crazy. People in this transition, people who are dying, often see things other people can't. It's perfectly natural. You don't have to be afraid or concerned."

His eyes dart around the room, tracking visions. Then, staring towards the foot of his bed, he whispers, "Who are you? There's a woman—her arms are crossed. She is looking down at me, beyond me. And who are *you?*" He mutters, staring straight up, his arms reaching up to the ceiling. Then, he dozes, with his arms still oddly reaching up toward the vision he's seen. When he awakens later, he looks at Barbara and me, his eyes welling, and cries out, "Oh, my darlings, oh my darlings, how I hate to leave you!"

Weeping, I put my arms around him, "Oh, Papa, I'll miss you so."

Barbara looks at him lovingly and says, "We've had a good 30 years together, more. We've been very lucky."

"Yes, yes we have," he replies. "What a story I could write. Wow! If only I could write this story …If I had the time …I'd begin with how lucky I am to have you with me at the end. …Oh, I could write this! What an opera it could be! What an opera."

Staring off as if writing the libretto and hearing the music, he drifts away again, clutching our hands. Abruptly, he wakes up a moment later, still holding our hands. Then he lets us go and with a resigned little chuckle, says, "I release you!"

Barbara and I glance at each other in wonder.

"Barbara," Dad says with a sweet smile, "I think this is the end. Please, Darling, don't leave the house anymore. I'm happy."

As he drifts back to sleep, Barbara turns to me with tears in her eyes, "He said he's happy."

"Yes, he did," I nod, heart full to bursting.

Standing at the foot of his bed while he sleeps later that day, I practice Chi Kung—the *Transition* form. With each move of the form, I whisper an affirmation, a prayer for his ease. Breathing out, "Papa, you can let go of your physical body." Breathing in, "Let the light in." Out, "Feel your wholeness." In, "Open space inside to allow this transformation." Out, "Become one with all that is." In, "Come home to your Source." Again and again, I practice, whispering words as I feel chi surge from the earth below and vibrate within me, emanating outward in circles around me, around his bed, around him.

During the days that follow, my father fluctuates back and forth between resisting and accepting his own death. One morning, he wakes up to the sound of the motion alarm. Panicked, he shouts out and Barbara and I come running. "What is it?" he asks urgently. "What's going on? It's a testing ground."

"No, Dear," Barbara assures him, "it's just the alarm."

"I'm being tested," Dad insists.

"What're you being tested for, Dad?"

"My resistance. It's my resistance."

"Resistance to what?"

"I don't know. I don't know." My father pauses. "Life's cruel."

"Yes, it is," Barbara agrees.

"Are you saying life's cruel because it ends?" I ask.

My father nods vehemently.

I muse softly, "Maybe that's a good thing. It's hard to let go of life, so perhaps that's why you think of it as cruel. I believe it's also beautiful, which may be why it is so hard to let go. It's good that you love being alive. I once read that our lives are a parenthesis in eternity. We come from eternity and return to it. I've often thought it was interesting that we're so afraid of what happens when we die, but we don't spend time being afraid of what was happening to us before we were born. I don't think we come in dreading life, perhaps we don't have to dread its end either."

"Babies cry," my father insists.

"What?" I ask.

"Babies come in crying. I came in crying, and I will leave wailing."

Barbara tells my father that she needs go to the kitchen to fix some supper. My father continues our conversation. "You know, it's really something to be at the end of my life and see what's really real."

"Yes," I reflect. "I think that may be a great gift that can come with the end of life."

His eyes widen, "Yes, yes, exactly, you're right. How do you know these things? How did you get to be so smart?"

"Look where I come from," I grin at him. Then I probe a bit further, "So what is it that you're finding is really real?"

He says, slowly, "My love for Barbara, and for you and the boys, and for certain pieces of my music. Not all of them. It's funny, I've written so many, but I only really care about a few."

"Which pieces?" I ask curiously. As a young man my father had considered becoming a priest, then became an atheist. Yet, in artistic contradiction to his beliefs, he won awards and fame not only for his operas, choral pieces, ballets, band music, and more, but also for his church music and orchestral pieces based on Gregorian themes. We talk about the pieces that are most important to him now.

"You know, for all I've done, it's really so small when you think of the multitude of music in the world."

"I think that could be said of any composer, Papa."

"Yeah, I guess…" His eyes cloud, then he turns to me bemused. "You know, I don't think I understand you. I've never seen…who you really are.

Tell me something—you seem so happy. You seem to be such a happy woman. What's your secret?"

I touch my chest, then his, and say, "I'd give you some if I could."

"No, I don't want it," he barks.

"Well," I muse, "I don't know for sure, but it's true I'm happy. I love my life and what it brings me."

"I just don't understand," he continues with his train of thought. "My God, every time you'd call, it's like everything would light up. The room would be brighter, like there was light all around."

Astonished, I say, "I had no idea, no idea you felt that way."

Looking lovingly at me, my father says, "I've been so mistaken about you. So much of my life, I just didn't like you. I'm so sorry. I didn't understand what you were, who you are. Now I know. I can see it. You're an angel. You are."

Days and nights go by. I awaken every morning at 5:00, stand outside my bedroom door on the landing just above my father's room, checking to hear the familiar sound of his snoring before beginning my hour meditation. Then I go outside to the back patio to greet the dawn with Chi Kung. The stillness of long hours waiting lulls me into an internal sense of spaciousness. Except for a few errands and some meals with Barbara, I spend most of my time in my father's room—reading, writing in my journal, or watching the leaves of the trees outside his window dance in the wind. Sometimes we talk, sometimes we simply hold eye contact, love exchanged with no words.

Days slip by, until one evening my father catches a second wind. "Ahhhhh! I can't stand it any longer. When's it gonna to be over? When'll it end? The waiting, this waiting …What the hell am I waiting for?!"

Sitting on his bed, I ask, "Are you hurting, Papa?"

Exasperated, my father shouts, "NO! It's just such a bore! Vic, can't you go get me a pill or something to make it be over? I want this to be over!"

"Do you mean a pill that would end your life?"

"Yes," he asserts. "This is horrible, just sleeping all the time. Make it stop. I want to stop!"

"I don't have a pill like that, Papa. But even if I did, I couldn't give it to you."

"Why?" he demands, irritated, then sardonic. "Are you afraid?"

"Well, yes, I am. Barbara and I would probably go to prison for a very long time. It's not legal to give someone a pill to help him die."

"Oh," he deflates. "But, why? Why is it like that? It's not right." His last bit of energy leaks out with a long sigh.

"It's not," I agree. "I think it's terrible that people can't make choices at the end of their lives about how they want to die. Uncle Ted felt like you on his last days. It's incredibly hard. But I do know that you can speed up this process if you stop eating and drinking. I promise you that either way this waiting will not go on forever, even though it seems like it will."

Later in the day, fumbling helplessly with his bedclothes, he says, "I can't find it. I had a card I was writing. I need to find it. I need to find it now."

"What were you writing?"

"My thoughts and wishes."

I look around a little. "I don't see any card here, but, if you'd like, I could go get my notebook and you can tell me what you've been writing and I'll transcribe it and read it back to you." Gratefully, he agrees.

When I sit down with my notebook and pen in hand, he begins. "I hope to come to the state where I would have the courage to end myself. If I could shut off my breath...but it's so hard to do ..."

I read back what he's said, and then ask, "Is that it?"

"No, not exactly. It's that it irks me to lie here and do nothing and not have the courage... It's not that I fear death, but what's painful is to think of doing something *against* myself. If you handed me something that would kill me immediately, I would do it, but actually killing myself is...I mean I am willing to kill myself, yet I'm afraid of doing it to myself. I'm such a coward."

I ask gently, "Are you afraid of your own cowardice?"

"Yeah, I dislike it immensely," he says as Barbara comes into the room. "Oh God, oh God, if only I had the courage to end this. If only I weren't such a coward!" Dad bursts out in a wail.

"I have a thought, Papa," I venture. "Maybe if instead of thinking of yourself as being a *coward* or *courageous*, you could change those words. Cowardice could become your *attachment to life*, and courage could be *letting go*. What if you imagined you are simply opening your fist? Your body is holding on so very tight, maybe you can imagine that it's slowly opening and letting go."

Barbara joins in, "Yes, that's right. That's a good way to think about it."

"Hmmm," he considers the possibility.

After my father decides to stop eating and drinking, his bodily functions slow down more rapidly and he slips into unconsciousness. I sit by him, stretch, and practice more Chi Kung in his room, doze in the little chaise placed near his bed. From time to time he moans, and I get up to whisper, "It's OK, Papa, I know you've worked really hard. Try to rest. It's almost over. Just relax and let go."

He does let go two days later. It is late afternoon when I notice his breathing has slowed down. Sometimes he takes a labored breath, then pauses for as much as 30 to 45 seconds before taking another. When he groans, I go to his bedside, hold his hand, stroke his head. This continues for hours. Then, abruptly, one of his eyes opens. I lean forward until I'm in his line of vision. I believe he can see me as we hold a gaze. His breathing slows even more, long gasps held for minutes. I place my hand on his chest over his heart. I call for Barbara.

When she comes in, I say, "Barbara, I think the time's very near now, and your face is the last thing he'd want to see." I draw her to where I have been standing, then step aside. Leaning forward with a little whimper, she places her hand on his, murmuring an endearment. His open eye locks on her. He takes a long, shuddering breath …a long pause …then another breath …a long pause, then one last breath. And his breathing stops. It is 7:05 p.m., ten days after I arrived.

Sitting next to his body on his bed, waiting for people from the funeral home, I said my goodbyes. I felt so happy that my father experienced the death he wanted, in his own bed, in his own house with Barbara and me by his side—the faces he'd said he wanted to see at the end. I had a deep sense of accomplishment that I somehow knew, just knew, the right moment to call for Barbara and, in so doing, fulfill my father's dying wish.

Like yang embedded in yin, I felt a kind of ecstasy inside my grief. Ecstasy in the profound sweetness wrought through changes activated by the integrity both of us experienced in coming back to the heart. I embraced the wholeness of this rocky journey made separately and together—the power and authenticity in our painful path to reconciliation.

As I look back on those days, I realize I took the *Way of Joy* with me, inside of me, and my father and I lived it together, our grief wedded to joy, our imminent separation filled with closeness, all old divisions melted into profound connection.

Our lives are complex, full of challenges, and we often don't know how to manage the many demands that fall upon us in even one day. The theory and practice of the *Way of Joy* is intended for both those ordinary days and the extraordinary ones as well. It is intended for spirals of growth and transformation that may take a moment in time or decades to accomplish fully. Even in the midst of life's complexities, my belief is that if you have a practice that empowers you to awaken inspiration, focus intention, and manifest fulfillment, you will be fueled by the infinite energy of joy.

APPENDIX

In my *Way of Joy* classes, I use information drawn from Traditional Chinese Medicine about the associations for the earth's respective seasons as a tool to assist students in mining the wisdom of their own internal "seasons" during the cycle of a year.

The Gifts of the Five Seasons

Because everything is in motion, all process is cyclic, and everything contains its opposite, the dilemma of what came first, the chicken or the egg, is transcended in Chinese philosophy by accepting them as inseparable agents of the process of creation. Chinese theory does not separate cause from effect; instead the one invariably turns into the other in an ever-repeating cycle of metamorphosis. The day does not cause the night, birth does not cause death, summer does not cause winter, but one precedes and the other follows. Life is a game of leapfrog with events tumbling over each other in a perpetual cascade. The chicken makes the egg—Yang generates Yin—but the chicken grows out of the egg—Yin produces Yang. They are only mutually generative. Which came first (linear logic) matters less than how they interact (systems, dialectical, relational logic).
— *Harriet Beinfield, L.Ac. and Efrem Korngold, L.Ac., O.M.D.*[1]

In Traditional Chinese Medicine (TCM), the body is regarded as a microcosm of the universe. Just as the natural world moves through daily and seasonal cycles, the body, mind/emotions and spirit also are in a constant state of cyclical change. Understanding the workings of the seasonal cycles, and the metaphors associated with them, is a fundamental way to grasp the Heaven aspect of the Earth triad. After all, the seasons and their corresponding weather are how we most directly experience the impact of Heaven on Earth, whether it be through the ferocious power of a raging blizzard, the welcome nourishment of spring rain, or the simple uplift of a sunny day. These seasonal cycles provide a context for the process of creation and manifestation.

The *Five Element* theory (also known as the *Five Phase* theory) is a system of thought within TCM that describes the process of transformation from one phase into another, the interrelationship and constraints of different elements that constitute balance.

The underlying assumption of Chinese philosophy is that the forces that govern the cycles of change occurring in the external world are duplicated within our human bodies and minds.

Patterns of nature are recapitulated at every level of organization—from the rotation of the planets to the behavior of our
internal organs. These ancient Oriental (*sic*) ideas conform to
what some modern thinkers call 'the holographic paradigm':
the organization of the whole (nature) is reflected by each and
every part (plants, animals, human beings).[2]

A comprehensive description of the Five Elements, their relationships and associations and the interplay between them, is beyond the scope
of this book.[3] My intention here is not to offer an explanation or even a
complete synopsis of this exquisitely complex worldview. Rather, I would
like to introduce you to a few basic concepts that may be helpful as you
consider your own life within the context of cycles. To do so, I have drawn
primarily from Mantak Chia's *Healing Tao*[4] system and from *Between Heaven
and Earth: A Guide to Chinese Medicine* by Beinfield and Korngold.[5]

Each of the seasons influences us both during the literal seasonal
time of year, and also by the characteristics of each season that can occur
at any time. Also associated with the seasons are the themes of birth,
growth, ripening, harvest, and decay.

I have found both in observing my students as well as in my own
practice that working with some of these Taoist themes can be extraordinarily helpful for connecting the microcosm of one's own consciousness
with that of a larger context, the macrocosm.

The *Five Phase* theory comprises five elements—metal, water, wood,
fire, and earth. Each of these corresponds to five seasons—the four seasons
plus a fifth season between summer and fall that is extended summer or
harvest (also known as "Indian Summer"). This fifth season corresponds to
the element of Earth and also represents a central balancing point, the transition between the seasons.

Just as the *Five Phases* delineate transformations of the life cycle,
they also describe the process of our daily existence. Our awakening is associated with *Wood*, and our movement toward a
state of compete wakefulness corresponds to *Fire*. Becoming
sleepy represents *Metal*, and the state of sleep itself corresponds
to *Water*. *Earth* represents the still point, the balance between
the polar movements, when neither one nor the other ascends.
Our integrity is based on the proportion and rhythm of each of
the *Five Phases* within us, regulating our waking and sleeping,
activity and rest, arousal and inhibition.[6]

The elements and seasons of the *Five Phase* system also correspond to different organs in your body—lungs, kidneys, liver, heart and stomach/spleen—as well as different emotions, including grief, fear, anger, hatred and anxiety.[7] Working to balance the five elements and all their associated components as expressed by the seasons is the key to maintaining optimal health and function.

The table below encapsulates some of the associations in the *Five Phase* system

Traditional Associations in the *Five Phase* System

	Spring	Summer	Late Summer	Autumn	Winter
Element	wood	fire	earth	metal	water
Direction	east	south	center	west	north
Time of Day	dawn	midday	late afternoon	dusk	midnight
Taste	sour	bitter	sweet	pungent*	salty
Sensory Organ	eyes	tongue	mouth, lips	nose**	ears***
Paired Organ	gall bladder	small intestine	stomach	large intestine	bladder
Color	green	red	yellow	white	blue
Animal	dragon	red pheasant	phoenix	white tiger	mule deer
Emotional Focus	transforming anger into kindness, forgiveness	transforming hatred and impatience into love and compassion	transforming worry and anxiety into balance and trust	transforming grief into courage	transforming fear into gentleness

* facilitates release through sweat – the skin is sometimes referred to as the third lung
** a primary conduit to the lungs
*** the better to listen to inner whisperings

In TCM, the seasons and elements not only cycle throughout the year, but also through our meridian systems on a daily basis. In fact, there are also specific hours where each meridian is activated and more dominant. Since each organ and its meridian is associated with a season, our bodies and psyches daily experience multi-leveled energetic cycles.

While I think it's vitally important to understand that our bodies are in a constant state of fluctuation and rebalancing, it's also important to not become too literal with this information. For example, if you're grieving the death of someone you love, you might well find that for a time your feelings of grief are the emotional backdrop for all other feelings. However, regardless of what you experience on a given day or moment, working with Chi Kung and meditation to balance and transform the dominant emotions will offer a sense of alignment with the greater forces at work, forces larger than your personal story. This in itself can provide comfort.

What follows is a brief synopsis of the seasonal cycles in terms of the energetic cycles of your body/spirit.[8]

Spring
Awaken from Winter's Stillness into the Tumultuous Emergence of New Life

Spring is the season when we bring forth seeds of the self that have been gestating during the winter. It is the time when your dreams are pushing to come forth and blossom. You may be looking for ways to refresh old visions, or you may have new flashes of inspiration that seem to come out of nowhere. Although many people associate Spring with light-hearted images of young love and butterflies, Spring is also a time of "emergenc-y," where your life force pushes forward unexpectedly and in potent ways. You may experience an internal sense of pressure as your second chakra energy of sexuality and creativity is activated. If you imagine a young tree as a pale seedling beginning to push through the winter-hardened earth, reaching for the warmth and light of the sun, you have an image for how insistent your own life force becomes during this point in your cycle.

In Taoist medicine, Spring is a time to cleanse, nourish and support your liver, which is associated with the element of Wood. Any suppressed feelings or intentions clamor to come forth. It is no surprise, then, that the emotion most often associated with the liver is anger. Just as it's not uncommon for a woman in childbirth to lash out in anger during the throes of labor, you may find the exhaustive work of your own "birthings" brings you to the same kind of emotional pitch. Within the vast interpretations of Chinese theory and medicine, I have found a variety of approaches that address the emotional aspects of the five elements. According to the teachings of Mantak Chia, when you move energy through your liver and break up stagnation, you transform anger into kindness and forgiveness. The movement from anger to forgiveness begins, I believe, with forgiveness of self. If you can move into the springtime of your cycle, whether it is actually Spring or not, with the intention to replace anger with kindness and forgiveness, you will return to the joy in your own creative process.

Metaphors for Spring
Planting, cultivating the soil, weeding, fertilizing, watering, tending, being with unfoldment, resistance versus strengthening, renewal, rebirth and birth.

Way of Joy **Focus for Spring**
Birthing new ideas and projects, nourishing what is coming forth, nurturing growth.

Summer
Open Gently to the Soul-Full Expression of Your Heart

Summer is the season when you experience your power in ways both vulnerable and strong as the seeds birthed in the Spring come to fruition. It is a time of flowering, heat and stillness, a time to allow the full expansion of your being to radiate from your heart.

The element of Summer is Fire, where you connect to the heat of your passion, to the things that matter most to you. The fires of summer flame into expression, maturation and expansion.

The Lotus Blossom is a metaphor for this season. In fact, there is a summer walking form of Chi Kung, inspired by that flower, which beautifully represents the energy and heart of this season. The thousand-petal lotus flower, a metaphor for enlightenment in many Eastern spiritual traditions, is rooted in the mud. Drawing nourishment from the seemingly stagnant and stinking ooze, the Lotus transforms that energy into a beautiful fragrance that wafts across the water. In the same way, during this season you are called upon to do the work of transforming the hardships and stagnation of the past into pure essential chi to open to the heart of your true being.

Dr. Quinn remarks that the word "flower" can be broken down to flow-er. "The secret of the flower," she says, "is that it knows how to flow gracefully within the seasons of its destiny."[9] To flow with the reality of all of our experiences, to translate stress into joy, is the work of the summer season.

Your heart is the home of impatience and hatred, the emotions that arise when you have felt blocked from your ability to care. Master Chia teaches that when you open energy in your heart, you change those painful emotions into Love and Compassion. Moving forward with the seeds of intention planted in the spring, summer is when you connect to both the autonomous individuality of your own personal passion and to others through community and interdependence. In full flower, the heart is the home to your joy. When you embrace this stage of your cycle, you flow in the world of possibility, of synchronicity, where you find yourself in the right place at the right time.

Metaphors for Summer

Tending, feeding, watering, empowerment, enjoyment, risking, telling the truth, opening to love, arranging flowers, creating beauty.

Way of Joy Focus for Summer

Expressing your passion, living your mastery, flowering into the full expression of your joy.

Extended or Late Summer (Indian Summer)
With an Easeful Breath, Rest into the Suspension between Seasons

At summer's end and before the onset of autumn, there is a time of lingering warmth, a final harvesting and relaxation as you transit from full expression to release. This is the time of "ripening, a stage during which we luxuriate in our maturity."[10] Corresponding to the element of Earth, this fifth season represents a time of balance and transition, opening space between the other four points in your cycle. In fact, in some depictions of the *Five Element* model, Earth resides at the center of the other four.

The organ associated with the season of Extended Summer and the element of Earth is the spleen.

> The spleen supplies the nourishment that sustains the organism. The raw material of food and experience is ingested, digested, and assimilated to fuel the life of the body and the mind...Like Mother Earth, the spleen is the constant provider, the hearth around which the body gathers to renew itself.[11]

As it is considered to be the balancing of the other four seasons and elements, Extended Summer is a time of transition, a period of letting go of what has been as you move into a new phase. Letting go can easily engender worry or anxiety, emotions associated with the spleen. As you prepare to move into autumnal release, you may find yourself wanting to hold on to what you accomplished in the last season of abundant expression. This time of maturity allows you to see how that expression may have influenced others, or be carried forth, as you prepare yourself for the contraction that inevitably follows expansion.

According to the *Healing Tao*, when you move energy through your spleen, you transform worry and anxiety to feelings of openness, fairness and faith. Trusting change as we move from one stage to the next, and viewing those changes as a part of a naturally occurring cycle, is key to balancing all of the emotions and staying connected to all-that-is.

Metaphors for Late Summer

Relishing maturity, transition, balance, trust, enjoying the harvest, suspending, accumulating wisdom.

Way of Joy Focus for Late Summer

Taking in what you have done, preparing yourself to let go, trusting in the ever-changing nature of life.

Autumn

In these Days and Nights of Deepening, Come Home to Your Essence

As the days grow shorter, the nights longer. Autumn is a time of letting go, releasing any excess, composting what you no longer need from what you may have achieved or accumulated during the summer. Fall teaches us to consolidate our energy in preparation for the cold months ahead.

In the Taoist tradition, Autumn is associated with Metal. Perhaps because I grew up in New York City, where buildings were always being torn down or constructed, I often envision the bare metal framework of high-rises before they are embellished with unique architectural façades. As metal constitutes the bare bones of the building, the Autumn point in the seasonal cycle represents the time when you access the bare bones of who you are, the core essence of your body/spirit.

Like a tree losing its leaves, this season represents a time of discernment and refinement, when you release your concerns about external circumstances and draw your attention inward to prepare for the long dreamtime of winter.

As you might imagine, the emotion associated with all of this release is grief. The primary organ associated with Autumn is the lungs. Just as the wind blows through tree branches, you might find yourself letting go of stress and pent-up energy with a big exhalation as you breathe through times of contraction and loss. The associated organ for Autumn (or the *Yang* partner of the *Yin* lungs) is the large intestine, another organ of letting go. Your large intestine rids your body of all the leftover waste material from which you extracted your nourishment. "By dispelling stale air and excreting turbid matter, the *Lung* and *Large Intestine* separate out that which we no longer desire or need."[12]

According to the practices of the *Healing Tao*, when you move energy through your lungs and breathe into the release of this season, you are cultivating your ability to transform grief into courage. Especially in a culture of acquisitiveness, I believe it does indeed entail courage to face loss on any level with the acceptance and grace that Nature so abundantly illustrates.

Metaphors for Autumn:
Pruning, releasing, letting go, balancing, contraction, discerning, self-regulation, making space, inner listening, remembering your core.

Way of Joy **Focus for Autumn**
Going to your core, listening for what is essential and true for you, for the qualities that have sustained you through your life.

Winter
Nourish Your Inner Flame as You Cradle Your Dreams

As the ground hardens and the air chills, we are drawn to go inside. Winter is the season when you are called to explore what lives below the surface, to pay attention to the internal workings of your psyche. Now is a time for rest and meditation so that you may replenish yourself as you listen to your dreams, the underground whisperings of the seeds of intention. "Before seeds and bulbs germinate, they demand a spell of chilly slumber."[13]

According to Taoist teachings, the element associated with Winter is Water. Often portrayed as a metaphor for the unconscious, Water is at the source of all life, pervading, adapting, sustaining.

Water is as subterranean as an underground stream, as dark and fertile as the womb, as enduring as the jade-colored sea. Water ascends to its fullness in the frost of winter as plants submerge their energy into their roots, animals thicken their hides, and ponds harden into ice. Movement slackens as matter and energy concentrate.[14]

Have you ever felt frozen with fear? Given all of the focus on the subterranean and the unconscious, it should be no surprise that the emotion associated with Water and Winter is fear. The experience of shaking that comes with a blast of fear is winter-y in its quality. When we go into the underworld, we inevitably encounter the faces of our demons, our buried terrors.

The organ associated with Winter and the element of Water is the kidneys, which regulate and balance water (and all other liquids) in our bodies. The associated organ is the bladder, which releases excess liquid. The kidneys, the seat of the adrenal glands, produce adrenaline, the chemical that creates the fight or flight response. Many practitioners recommend that you be sure to keep your kidneys warm because it's vital to keep the inner flame of your consciousness burning and sustaining your intention.

According to the *Healing Tao*, when you send chi through your kidneys, you transform fear into gentleness. In fact, the animal association in this particular system is the mule deer, a small animal that seems the epitome of gentleness. When you have a dream of being pursued, like a deer being hunted, it is often recommended that you as the dreamer turn to face the fears that are chasing you. When you do, you usually find new understandings waiting to be seen and acknowledged. This creates a shift of consciousness, from which gentleness in the face of your own fear can ensue.

This kind of fluid adaptability, the transformation of fear into gentle compassion, is like that of water, which can change into a myriad of forms from a raging river or to a delicate crystalline snowflake.

Metaphors for Winter
Hibernating, dreaming, facing demons, sustaining, waiting, stockpiling resources, going to the roots, moistening.

Way of Joy Focus for Winter
Listening to your dreams, resting and replenishing, traveling into the depths of your own consciousness, adapting, transforming.

A SELECTED BIBLIOGRAPHY

Anandamoy, Bro. Taped Lecture, "The Liberating Power of Affirmation," based on *The Divine Romance* by Paramahansa Yogananda. Given at the Self-Realization Fellowship, Pasadena, CA. For more information, call (323) 225-2471.

Beinfeld, Harriet and Efrem Korngold. *Between Heaven and Earth: A Guide to Chinese Medicine.* New York: Ballantine Books, 1991.

Cameron, Julia. *The Artist's Way: A Spiritual Path to Higher Creativity.* New York: Tarcher/Putnam, 1992.

Cameron, ———. *The Vein of Gold: A Journey to Your Creative Heart.* New York:Putnam, 1996.

Capra, Fritjof. *The Tao of Physics (4th edition).* Boston: Shambala Publications,1999.

Chen, Nancy N. *Breathing Spaces: Qigong, Psychiatry and Healing in China.* New York: Columbia University Press, 2003.

Cheng Man-Ch'ing and Robert Smith, *T'ai-Chi: The Supreme Ultimate Exercise for Health, Sport, and Self-Defense.* Rutland: Charles E. Tuttle, Co., 1974.

Chopra, Deepak. "What is the True Nature of Reality? The Basics of Quantum Healing." *Harmony* on-line magazine. Web address: http://manifestingmindpower.com/deepakchopra.htm.

Dewey, Reiko Myamoto. Interview with Masuro Emoto. *The Spirit of Maat* on-line magazine. Web address: http://www.spiritofmaat.com/archive/nov1/cwater.htm.

Dyer, Wayne. *The Power of Intention: Learning to Co-Create Your World Your Way.* Carlsbad: Hay House, Inc., 2004.

Dispenza, Joe, D.C. *Evolve Your Brain: The Science of Changing Your Mind.* Deerfield Beach: Health Communications, Inc., 2007.

Ellison, Sharon. *Taking the War Out of Our Words: The Art of Powerful, Non-Defensive Communication.* Deadwood: Wyatt-MacKenzie Publishing, 1998.

Emoto, Masaru. *The Hidden Messages in Water.* Trans. David A. Thayne. Hillsboro: Beyond Words, 2004.
Goldman, Caren. On-line interview with Dr. Candace Pert. Web address: http://www.leonieslight.org/view_article.asp?id=245.

Hanh, Thich Nhat. *Touching Peace: Practicing the Art of Mindful Living.* Berkeley: Parallax, 1992.

Harris, Bill. *Thresholds of the Mind: Your Personal Roadmap to Success, Happiness, and Contentment.* Beaverton: Centerpointe Press, 2007.

Hawkins, David R., M.D., Ph.D. *Power vs. Force: The Hidden Determinants of Human Behavior.* Carlsbad: Hay House, 2002.

Hintz, J, Yount, G, Kadar I, Schwartz G, Hammerschlag R, Lin S. "Bioenergy definitions and research guidelines." *Altern Ther Health Med 9* (3 Suppl), 2003.

Houston, Jean. On-line interview with James Twyman. Web address: http://www.freetelemessages.com/programs.cfm?id=184.

Kornfield, Jack. *A Path With Heart: A Guide Through the Perils and Promises of Spiritual Life.* New York: Bantam Books, 1993.

Lefer, Diane. "The Blessing is Next to the Wound: A Conversation with Hector Aristizábal About Torture and Transformation." *The Sun.* October, 2005.

LeGuin, Ursula, transl. Lao Tzu. *Tao Te Ching: The Book About the Way and the Power of the Way.* Boston: Shambala Publications, 1997.

Leonard, George and Michael Murphy. *The Life We Are Given: A Long-Term Program for Realizing the Potential of Body, Mind, Heart and Soul.* New York: Tarcher/Penguin Books, 2005.

Lipton, Bruce. *The Biology of Belief: Unleashing the Power of Consciousness, Matter & Miracles.* Carlsbad: Hay House, 2005.

Logan, William Bryant. *Dirt: The Ecstatic Skin of the Earth.* New York: Riverhead Books, 1995.

MacRitchie, James. *Chi Kung: Energy for Life.* London: Thorsons, 2002.

Mayer, Michael, Ph.D. "Qigong and Behavioral Medicine: An Integrated Approach to Chronic Pain." *Qi—The Journal of Traditional Health and Fitness.* Winter 1996-1997.

Mitchell, Stephen, transl. Lao Tzu. *Tao Te Ching.* New York: Harper & Row, 1988.
Myss, Caroline, Ph.D. *Anatomy of the Spirit: The Seven Stages of Power and Healing.* New York: Three Rivers Press, 1996.

Naff, Monza, Ph.D. *Exultation: A Poem Cycle in Celebration of the Seasons.* Deadwood: Wyatt-MacKenzie Publishing, 1999.

Naff, ———. *Healing the Womanheart.* Deadwood: Wyatt-MacKenzie Publishing, 1999.

Padma, Ma Deva. *Tao Oracle: An Illuminated New Approach to I Ching* (cards and book). New York: St. Martin's Press, 2002.

Quinn, Khaleghl, Dr. *Chi Kung: Reclaim Your Power: The Secret Art of Maximizing Your Potential.* Northhampton: Thorsons (Harper Collins), 1995.

Quinn, ———. *Everyday Self-Defense: Protect Yourself with Attitude, Intuition, and Strategy.* San Francisco: Harper Collins, 1994.

Quinn, ———. *Khaleghl Quinn's Art of Self-Defense.* Northhampton: Thorsons (Harper Collins), 1993.

Quinn, ———. *Stand Your Ground.* London: Oribs Publishing Ltd., 1983.

Tolle, Eckart. *A New Earth: Awakening to Your Life's Purpose.* New York: Plume, 2006.

Ueshiba, Morihei. Web address: http://www.aikiweb.com/general/memoir.html.

Wilber, Ken. *Grace and Grit: Spirituality and Healing in the Life and Death of Treya Killam Wilber.* Boston: Shambhala, 2000.

FOOTNOTES

Note to Reader
[1] James MacRitchie, *Chi Kung: Energy for Life* (London: Thorsons, 2002), p. 9.
[2] Nancy N. Chen, *Breathing Spaces: Qigong, Psychiatry and Healing in China* (New York: Columbia University Press, 2003), p. 6.

Prologue
[1] To learn more about Dr. Quinn's work and teachings, please visit her websites: www.lotusbeing.com and www.atarainstitute.com.
[2] In martial arts, a belt test is an exam given to mark a progression in rank of ability.

Chapter One
[1] This concept is also consistent with Dr. Quinn's teachings of the *Lotus*, a Seasonal Tonic Chi Kung form, where she describes joy as "the ability to feel and express the full spectrum of emotions."

Chapter Two
[1] For this story, as well as other stories in the book, except for those who have given me permission, I have changed the names of the people involved to protect their privacy.
[2] Kajukenbo is a hybrid martial art developed in Hawaii by several different black belts who incorporated their different martial arts styles to respond to increasing street violence.
[3] Wayne Dyer, *The Power of Intention: Learning to Co-Create Your World Your Way* (Carlsbad: Hay House, Inc., 2004), p. 14.
[4] The metaphor of compost is used in Khaleghl Quinn's teaching of Chi Yoga.
[5] *Power of Intention.* p. 188.
[6] Some of the characteristics in Charts 2 and 3 such as Wisdom—Joy—Health/Wealth, and Inspiration, Love and Manifestation, come from the Three Gates of Enlightenment, one of the seminal forms of Chi Kung Dr. Quinn references in *Reclaim Your Power.* pp. 35-44. The artwork for these charts was done by Sherry Mouser. www.mouserart.com.

Chapter Three
[1] *Touching Peace: Practicing the Art of Mindful Living* (Berkeley: Parallax,1992), pp.1-2.

Chapter Four
[1] *Tao Oracle: An Illuminated New Approach to I Ching.* (New York: St. Martin's Press, 2002), p. 61.
[2] For more information, visit www.pndc.com.
[3] *Tao Oracle,* p. 60.
[4] I first heard this term from Dr. Quinn when studying the *Lotus* with her.
[5] The 1983 movie, *Koyaanisqatsi,* based on the Hopi word signifying a world out of balance, depicts the danger of unending expansion on a global level. Using only

imagery and music, the film vividly portrays the unrelenting pursuit of industrial production and the impact it has on the environment, as the planet is pillaged for resources and Nature is commodified. The visuals of this powerful film have stayed with me all these years and have become a part of my foundation for understanding the global impact of living out of balance with Nature.

[6] From an online interview with Reiko Myamoto Dewey for *The Spirit of Maat* http://www.spiritofmaat.com/archive/nov1/cwater.htm.

[7] This quote is from a taped lecture, *The Liberating Power of Affirmation,* given at the Self Realization Fellowship in Pasadena, Ca. For more information, you may call 323-225-2471.

Chapter Five

[1] (kidney 1 point, located in the hollow below the center of the ball of the foot)

[2] In her inspiring book, *Reclaim Your Power,* which I highly recommend, the *Shower* is the third in a series of short exercises that Dr. Khaleghl Quinn calls "Chi Cybernetics." I have included three other short forms from this series—the *Fountain, Pump,* and *Pebble in the Lake*—in future Practice chapters. Original creations of Dr. Quinn, these particular exercises and their concurrent teachings were developed out of her observations of repetitive themes within the fluid Chi Kung forms, as well as concepts within Zen, Kung Fu and other systems. For the *Way of Joy* Practices in this book, I've received permission from the author to use four exercises that embody some of the themes within the three Practices. Please see her original book for more information.

[3] The phrase "Steeping the Tea" was coined by Dr. Khaleghl Quinn. The techniques for both Steeping the Tea and Tapping come from her teachings of Chi Yoga. The final "sweep and splash" movement from *Tapping It In* is a technique she created to integrate flow around the Microcosmic Orbit.

Part Two

[1] Ken Wilber, *Grace and Grit: Spirituality and Healing in the Life and Death of Treya Killam Wilber* (Boston: Shambhala, 2000), p. 304.

Chapter Six

[1] Cheng Man-Ch'ing and Robert Smith, *T'ai-Chi: The Supreme Ultimate Exercise for Health, Sport, and Self-Defense* (Rutland: Charles E. Tuttle, Co., 1974), p. 5.

[2] Physicist Amit Goswami, Ph.D, in *What the Bleep Do We Know?*, a Lord of the Wind film, William Arntz, Betsy Chasse, Mark Vicente, producers, 2004.

[3] in *What the Bleep Do We Know?* William Tyler is also author of the book, *Conscious Acts of Creation.*

[4] Deepak Chopra, "What is the True Nature of Reality? The Basics of Quantum Healing." *Harmony* on-line magazine. http://manifestingmindpower.com/deepak-chopra.htm.

[5] Michael Mayer, Ph.D., "Qigong And Behavioral Medicine: An Integrated Approach To Chronic Pain," *Qi —The Journal of Traditional Eastern Health and Fitness.* Winter 1996-1997, p 23.

[6] J Hintz, G Yount, I Kadar, G Schwartz, R Hammerschlag, S Lin, "Bioenergy defini-tions and research guidelines." *Altern Ther Health Med 9* (3 Suppl), 2003, A13-30.

[7] Ibid.

[8] Webpage: http://www.aikiweb.com/general/memoir.html.

[9] Deepak Chopra, "What is the True Nature of Reality?" *Harmony* on-line magazine. http://manifestingmindpower.com/deepakchopra.htm.

[10] *Tao Oracle*, p. 97.

[11] *Grace and Grit*, p. 304.

Chapter Seven

[1] Dojo, workout studio

[2] In her brilliant model of *Powerful Non-Defensive Communication*™, Sharon Ellison (www.pndc.com) theorizes that every word we use is a blueprint that contains within it what she calls a VERB element: V=value, E= emotion, R = reasoning, B = behavior. She describes how these blueprints define our reality.

[3] You can learn more about Sharon Strand Ellison's theories, work, and products including her book, *Taking the War Out of Our Words: The Art of Powerful Non-Defensive Communication,* on her website www.pndc.com.

Chapter Eight

[1] Sharon Ellison, *Taking the War Out of Our Words: The Art of Powerful, Non-Defensive Communication* (Berkeley: Bay Tree Publishing, 2002), p. 235.

[2] *The Artist's Way: A Spiritual Path to Higher Creativity* (New York: Tarcher/Putnam, 1992), p. 3.

[3] *Reclaim Your Power.* p. 148.

[4] I first learned the concept of *wei chi* from Dr. Quinn.

[5] *Reclaim Your Power.* p. 131. The *Fountain* is the second "Chi Cybernetic."

[6] This practice can be greatly augmented for interpersonal communication when used in conjunction with the communication tools defined in Sharon Ellison's work in *Powerful Non-Defensive Communication.* www.pndc.com

[7] This Chi Kung healing practice by Jarboux can also be found in the anthology by James MacRitchie, *Chi Kung: Energy for Life.* (London: Thorsons, 2002), p.140.

[8] You will find *Align Heaven and Earth Level 1* in the *Stance Preparation* earlier in this chapter.

[9] This part of the exercise "what *do* I want?" is adapted from exercises and sugges-tions I have encountered in my work with Life Coach Dory Willer and in a teleconference course with author Michael Losier, both practitioners of the Law of Attraction.

Part Three

[1] Harriet Beinfield and Efrem Korngold, *Between Heaven and Earth: A Guide to Chinese Medicine* (New York, Ballantine Books, 1991), p. 29. [2] *Evolve Your Brain* (Deerfield Beach: Health Communications, Inc.), 2007, p. 3.

[3] Caroline Myss, Ph.D., *Anatomy of the Spirit: The Seven Stages of Power and Healing* (New York: Three Rivers Press, 1996), p. 61.

[4] Lefer, "The Blessing is Next to the Wound: A Conversation with Hector Aristizábal About Torture and Transformation" *The Sun* (October, 2005), pp. 5-7.

Chapter Nine
[1] *Between Heaven and Earth*, p. 29.
[2] For a more in-depth discussion about the meanings associated with the seasons in Traditional Chinese Medicine, please see Appendix.
[3] Artist/healer, this is my good friend who died that I mentioned in my Prologue and Chapter 4.
[4] For information about how to ask questions that disarm power struggle, whether externally with others or internally in your psyche, see Sharon Ellison's work at www.pndc.com.
[5] I again recommend that you look at Ellison's work with *Powerful Non-Defensive Communication,* which presents valuable guidance on how to make empowered statements and set clear limits.
[6] Joe Dispenza, D.C., *Evolve Your Brain: The Science of Changing Your Mind* (Deerfield Beach: Health Communications, Inc., 2007), p. 46.

Chapter Ten
[1] Tigunait, "How to Live a Truly Joyful Life." *Yoga+Joyful Living.* July-August, 2006, p. 33.
[2] *Tao Oracle.* P. 256
[3] Online interview with Caren Goldman
http://www.leonieslight.org/view_article.asp?id=245.
[4] Lipton, *The Biology of Belief: Unleashing the Power of Consciousness, Matter & Miracles* (Carlsbad, Hay House, 2005). His lectures on CD are also profoundly illuminating.
[5] Stephen Mitchell, transl. Lao Tzu. *Tao Te Ching* (New York: Harper & Row, 1988), p. 23.
[6] Leonard and Murphy, *The Life We Are Given: A Long-Term Program for Realizing the Potential of Body, Mind, Heart and Soul.* (New York: Tarcher/Penguin Books, 2005), p. 47.
[7] Jack Kornfield, *A Path With Heart: A Guide Through the Perils and Promises of Spiritual Life.* (New York: Bantam Books, 1993), p. 108.
[8] Wilber, *Grace and Grit.* (Boston: Shambhala, 2000), p. 250.
[9] On-line interview with James Twyman,
http://www.freetelemessages.com/programs.cfm?id=184.

Chapter Eleven
[1] Harris, *Thresholds of the Mind: Your Personal Roadmap to Success, Happiness, and Contentment* (Beaverton: Centerpointe Press, 2007), p. 94. Note: Founder of the Centerpointe Research Institute and creator of a brilliant audio technology he calls Holosync that balances the right and left hemispheres of the brain to induce deep meditation, Bill Harris provides a comprehensive approach on how to better understand the workings of our unconscious and what he calls the "nuts and bolts" of how we manifest in our lives and create our own reality. Visit his website at http://www.centerpointe.com.

[2] These next two practices come from Dr. Quinn's stretch routine.

[3] These are both practices I learned from Dr. Khaleghl Quinn. *Transition* is drawn from a longer set of Flowing Forms.

[4] Quinn, *Reclaim Your Power*, p. 119.

[5] For both this exercise and the *Lotus Push*, I have drawn upon the longer seasonal summer form the *Lotus*, which I originally studied with Dr. Quinn.

[6] You can read more about Emoto's work and the principle of *Hado* on the web at www.hado.net or in his book, *The Hidden Messages of Water.*

[7] A highly developed system, "Voice Dialogue" itself is beyond the scope of this book You can get more information from the founders, Drs. Stone, on their website at http://www.delos-inc.com. This exercise is my own personal exploration inspired by the concept of "Voice Dialogue" as I understand it and is not meant to be a representation of their work.

Chapter Twelve

[1] Lyrics for a choral piece, *A Jubilant Song*, by my father, Norman Dello Joio, adapted from *A Song of Joys* by Walt Whitman.

Appendix

[1] *Between Heaven and Earth: A Guide to Chinese Medicine* (New York: Ballantine Books, 2001), p. 51. This is one of my favorite books on Chinese Medicine.

[2] Ibid., p. 87.

[3] There are hundreds of books available that describe the *Five Element* theory in much more depth. You'll find a wealth of information in books on Traditional Chinese Medicine.

[4] Mantak Chia is the founder of the *Healing Tao* and author of many books of Taoist philosophy, meditation practices and Chi Kung.

[5] *Between Heaven and Earth* also includes questionnaires for self-evaluation to explore your personal dominant characteristics within this complex cosmology.

[6] Ibid., p. 89.

[7] Other associations with colors, tastes, senses, animals and so on can be found in any book on Chinese medicine or the *Five Element* theory.

[8] An extraordinary exploration of the meanings of the seasons and what we can learn from them can be found in Monza Naff's poem cycle, *Exultation*, available in book form or on CD that includes guided meditations. See www.pndc.com.

[9] *Reclaim Your Power,* p. 11.

[10] Ibid., p. 89.

[11] Ibid., p. 112.

[12] Ibid., p. 120.

[13] Ibid., p.218.

[14] Ibid., p 218.

INDEX OF CHARTS AND TABLES

These charts and tables are available for download and printing (some in color) at www.wayofjoy.com/resources

INDEX OF EXERCISES

Meditations: Illuminating

Heaven

Human

Earth

Life Observation Exercises for Accessing:

Heaven

Human

Earth

Journal Exercises: Deepening

Heaven

Human

Earth

GENERAL INDEX

R

Reality
  creating it, 214
  forces beyond our control, Taoist
    Tale, farmer and son, 215
  self-blame for conditions we can't
    change, Arthur, 215
  co-creating reality, mystery and
    complexity, 216, 217
  reality dissolved, possibility, limit
    less, Vicki, Wolfgang, 220
Reciprocity, 62, 140, 141
Reconciliation, Vicki and her father
  setting boundaries after he
    disowned her, 139, 140
  overcoming intimidation to full
    empowerment, 266-271
  father's death process, accounta
    bility, clarity, love, 271-277
Resistance *see acceptance*
  self-examination, Kevin, critical
    mother, 185
  resistance to transition, 191
  moving out of resistance into
    insight, 192-198
  constructive and destructive uses of
resistance, 212
  role of resistance, keeping integrity
    with values, 213
  resistance in the face of empower
    ment, 226
  getting stronger, near manifestation,
    227
Roethke, Theodore, 179
Rhiannon, 132

S

Sarton, May, 55
Secret, The, 214
Self-Esteem
  inflated ego, 70
  deflated ego, 71
  balanced ego, 72
  healthy boundaries a key to self-
    esteem, 143, 144
  reclaiming discernment, Carla 145-
    147
  self-esteem versus modesty, Vicki,
    148
  writer who gave up writing, 148,
    149

Shange, Ntozake, 115
Six Healing Sounds, 250
Space
  space between, time out, 119
  space in our bodies, 121
  space in solid matter, Kajukenbo,
    breaking boards, Vicki, 122
  moving chi in the space between,
    boards and stones, 122, 125
  space, empty or full, 126
  source of creativity, 125, 126
  inner space and universal
    consciousness, 127
  boundaries define space, 137
Spiral, Downward *see circles, pivoting*
  stagnation leads to downward
spiral, 187
  rock bottom, 192
  offers useful information, 191
Spiral, Upward
  from circle to outward spiral, 190
  facing conflict, Manuel and boss,
    195-197
Spirituality, 140, 141-143
Steinbeck, John, 199
Stillness
  empty mind, surfing, Lucinda, 45
  empty mind, Kajukenbo, Reba, 45
  internal, during external chaos, 47,
    48
  how stillness saved my life, hit by a
    car, Vicki, 51
Stone, Hal and Sidra, Drs., 259
Stress
  breath, stillness in motion during
    external chaos, Manuel, 48
  stagnant energy, 120

T

Taking the War Out of Our Words, 148
Tao Oracle, 55
Tao Te Ching
  quote, 117
  23rd Verse, 210
Taoism and Taoist Philosophy
  definition, ix
  realms, 30
  old Taoist text, 44
  opposites, complementary, 55
  healing, 123
  Taoist Tale, farmer and son, 215

AUTHOR BIOGRAPHY

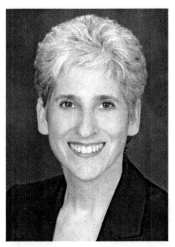

Vicki Dello Joio is a Master Teacher of Chi Kung, a seasoned theater performer and director, speaker, and consultant. Vicki is a member of the faculty at John F. Kennedy University and a master trainer of *Powerful Non-Defensive Communication™*. In 1994, she founded the *Way of Joy* Center where she offers workshops and classes to the public.

A graduate of Sarah Lawrence College, Vicki has extensive training with master teachers, including Tai Chi Master Franklin Kwong, Ed Young from Master Cheng Man-Ch'ing's school in New York, and Chi Kung Master Khaleghl Quinn in California. Vicki studied theater arts at Carnegie-Mellon University and at Hagen-Berghoff Studio with Herbert Berghoff. She learned the Feldenkreis Method from Katya Delakova, an early student of Moshe Feldenkreis. She studied mime in Paris with Etienne Decroux, teacher of Marcel Marceau, and physical theater with Jacques Le Coq, founder of the L'Ecole Internationale de Theater Jacques Lecoq.

Vicki co-founded, directed and performed with Common Threads Theatre Company, which toured for seven months in Europe. She choreographed *Synergy*, a work commissioned for the company by the American Association of University Women, performed at the Moscone Center in San Francisco. Vicki also appeared in a critically acclaimed one-woman show, *A Mime's Eye View*.

Vicki is a member of the Living Arts Playback Theatre Ensemble which performs publicly, at national conferences, and with the Healing the Wounds of History project, which brings together polarized groups such as African-Americans and European-Americans and Palestinians and Israelis, to transform the pain of shared historical legacies into constructive action.

With her diverse background, Vicki has developed unique teaching methods that empower people to focus their energy with increased awareness, transforming obstacles into opportunities and enhancing their creative potential. She has been a presenter at many conferences and organizations, including the National Qigong Association, martial arts and yoga schools across the country, as well other professional and community organizations such as Saint Joseph Regional Medical Center and the Oakland Museum.

As a facilitator, Vicki's presentations include interactive dialogue, theater games, and martial arts as teaching tools with a wide range of applications for personal growth, professional development and community building. Her speeches and workshops have proven highly effective for leadership development, conflict resolution, and communication across cultural differences.

Contact Vicki Dello Joio: **Web:** www.wayofjoy.com **Email:** Vicki@wayofjoy.com

LaVergne, TN USA
30 December 2009

168571LV00003B/2/P

9 780982 051894